Come Alive!

50 Easy Ways to Have More Energy Now

Karen Rowinsky

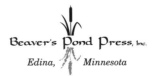

Beaver's Pond Press, Inc.

Edina, Minnesota

ISBN 1-890676-79-9

Library of Congress Catalog Number: 00-108549

Printed in the United States of America.

03 02 01 00   5 4 3 2 1

*For my dad,
the late Philip Schuss,
who taught me how to work,
and my mom, Maralyn Levine,
who taught me how to play,
loving thanks for these
equally important gifts.*

Table of Contents

Acknowledgements

*M*y life has been blessed in a multitude of ways, most importantly by the people in it. Their love and support have made the hard times easier and the good times better. To the thousands of women and men who have attended my "Energizing" presentations over the last ten years, I thank you for your smiling faces and the many ideas you have shared.

To my friends and readers: Nicole Basso, Elizabeth Blanchard, Alice Cnossen, Madeline Finch, Pola Firestone, Shirley Garrett, Nancy Hedrick, Mary O'Brien, Deborah Shouse, Barbara Shapiro, and Stephanie Snyder, thanks for your kind words and thoughtful comments. I appreciated your honesty and the time and energy you gave to help me achieve my dream. To my Master Mind group, thank you for your gentle encouragement and for holding me accountable.

To Milt Adams and the folks at Beaver's Pond Press, Connie Anderson, and Jack Caravela thanks for your patience and support as I gave birth to my dream. I didn't realize it was almost as challenging as giving birth to a real baby. To my National Speakers Association friends, you are my teachers and role models. Thank you for embracing me (literally) and showing me the possibilities.

Thank you and hugs to my "soul sisters" Billie Hall, Leslie Jenison, Mary O'Brien, and Jeanie Smith and my "soul brother" J. Schafer. Your spirit has fed mine and I am forever grateful that you are in my life. To my friend and guide, Mark LeBlanc, thank you for your enthusiasm and brilliant ideas which have made my work come alive! To my friend and advisor Katherine Kent, one of the wisest women I know, thank you for the common sense words and ideas that found their way into my head and my heart.

To Katie and Valerie Gumpertz, thanks for teaching me how to be a stepmom and for generously sharing your dad. To my daughter Alissa, and my son Daniel, you have filled my life with magical moments. Thank you for your love and patience as I learned how to be your mom. Even when life was incredibly hard for us, you gave me the energy I needed to keep walking my talk.

And to my husband, friend, and partner Rick Gumpertz, I can only hope that you know the depth of my gratitude to you for coming into my life and for the love and delight you brought with you. You were definitely worth the wait!

Karen Rowinsky

Introduction

*I*n my previous career, I designed and implemented community education programs for a hospital women's health center. In several classes a month, I helped women and men learn how to live healthier, more satisfying lives. The evaluation form for these programs questioned, "What would you like to know to help you lead the life you want?" The most frequent reply was, "I want to find a way to have more energy."

Like these people, I too, had more things to do each day than my energy allowed. Worse than that, I didn't seem to have one spare minute to find more energy. I needed a quick fix now, not a life style change or long-term solutions with results to come some time in the future. So, I set about researching ways people can achieve more energy without putting much of their precious energy into attaining it. The strategies in this book are the result of that research.

Even though finding more energy is a matter of common sense, we sometimes don't use our common sense when we are feeling tired and drained. While some aspects of these strategies require more time than others, each one has an "Energizing Tip" that can yield results apparent right away. With that boost, you will have the added energy to go on to explore additional strategies.

We all have different needs, desires, interests, and strengths. I believe that after reading this book that compiles the 50 best strategies I've collected, you will find many that will work for you. Have an open mind and try as many as possible. But, don't do them all at one time. That definitely would defeat the purpose of having more energy!

E-mail or write me the strategies that work for you and tell what was effective, how you might have embellished a particular strategy or best of all, what new strategies I should add to this collection to benefit others.

I believe each of us can have more energy. The amount is relative to the time in your life, the circumstances in which you live, and your health. If you want more energy, you can have it. The choice is yours!

Karen Rowinsky
Come Alive!
P.O. Box 11606
Shawnee Mission, Kansas 66207
Karen@50EasyWays.com
www.50EasyWays.com

Karen Rowinsky

Part One:

Getting Started

*I*t may be easy to say the choice is yours to have more energy. Realistically, it can be challenging to take control and make that choice. By choosing to add more energy to our lives, we are committing ourselves to breaking habits we may have had for a very long time. Feeling sluggish, inert, or tired is sometimes just a bad habit. Making the decision to change this habit may be invigorating enough to give you what you need to take that first step.

No matter how healthy or happy we are, there will always be a time when we wish we had more energy. Each stage of our life offers opportunities for energy drain. Whether you are in your 20s, 30s, 70s, 80s, or anywhere in between, you will probably experience low energy at some point in each day. This book is for those times.

Most adults know that if they maintain a healthy weight, exercise regularly, eat a nutritional diet, have healthy relationships, and enjoy good mental health, then they will have more energy. If you are like most of us though, there are certain times in your life, you do not or cannot live optimally. Does that mean your energy is an all-or-nothing proposition? Absolutely not!

The strategies in this book are divided into the three ways you may experience energy or the lack of it. You will find ways to renew, refresh, and reinvigorate your body, mind, and spirit.

Each is an integral part of who we are and each offers us many opportunities to add energy to our life.

Let's get to it!

What Does It Feel Like to Have All the Energy You Want?

*D*o you remember a time in your life when you had all the energy you wanted or needed? I've found that experiencing what that felt like will help you incorporate energizing strategies into your life now. Try the following exercise to help you remember what it felt like. (You may want to enlist the help of someone who can read the exercise out loud while you do it. Or read through it before you begin and try to remember the specific steps.)

Sit relaxed in a comfortable chair. Clear your mind by closing your eyes and begin concentrating on your breathing. Breathe in deeply through your nose and let it out your mouth. Breathe as slowly as comfortable, counting to four as you inhale and again as you exhale. Repeat.

Think about the time when you last felt that you had all the energy you needed. You probably weren't even aware of your energy level: It was just there. You may have to go back a couple of years, a couple of decades, or more, but remember that time and begin to see yourself living in it.

Try to picture where you lived then. Who did you live with? What did your house or apartment look like? What did your room look like? If that memory is far back in time, picture the fashions of the day. What kind of music was popular? Can you remember a particular song you liked?

Now remember yourself on a typical day. What might you be doing? See yourself doing those activities. Take a minute and examine how you feel. You are remembering a time when you had all the energy you wanted or needed. Enjoy the sensations for a few minutes.

- How does your body feel?
- What kind of sensations are you experiencing?
- What about your mind?
- How does your thinking differ from when you are feeling drained?
- What about the spirit within you?
- What kind of mood are you in?

Now return to the present. Do it slowly. Become aware of your breathing. Take a few deep breaths in through your nose and let them out your mouth. To ease the transition back to the present, become aware of the air on your skin. Before you open your eyes, picture the room you are in. Then just relax for a few minutes after opening your eyes.

After this time travel, you are ready to put your experiences to use. Take a piece of paper and write down some words that describe how you felt when you went back and experienced having all the energy you wanted or needed. Make a list describing how your body and mind felt. Describe your mood or the spirit within you.

To get you started, you might review the following words that others have used to describe the sensation of feeling energized:

Body: Light, bouncy, good, bubbly, free, breathe easier, comfortable, floating, tingly

Mind: Clear thinking, have good memory, optimistic, positive, resourceful, creative

Spirit: Happy-go-lucky, enthusiastic, spirited, increased sense of humor, loving, excited

Wow! Who wouldn't want to have more energy if they felt like that? Keep the list of words as an incentive or reminder of your mission to build more energy into your life.

If you are so revved up that you don't want to waste another minute before getting started, turn to some of the strategies. Try one or two that appeal to you. For most, however, I would recommend completing the following quiz to determine what zaps your energy. The results can better direct your choice of strategy. For overall, long-lasting success this step is well worth it.

What Drains Your Energy?

*B*efore picking a strategy more or less at random, figure out what drains the energy from you. Take the following quiz to identify which area or areas of your life might be depleting your energy.

In the blank to the left of each statement write the number that best describes your behavior:

3=Always, 2=Most of the time, 1=Sometimes, 0=Never

BODY	
____	I exercise 30 minutes four to five times per week.
____	I eat a healthy, balanced diet.
____	I drink at least 8 eight-ounce glasses of water a day.
____	I get enough sleep each night to wake refreshed.
____	I see my health care provider regularly and receive health screening tests when these are indicated.
____	Total

MIND	____ I rarely hold grudges or stay angry at people.
	____ I rarely overextend myself or make too many commitments.
	____ I choose what I want to do and can easily say no.
	____ I value lifelong learning and seek opportunities to use my mind.
	____ I am organized at home and at work and rarely lose or forget things that are important to me.
	____ Total
SPIRIT	____ I take time every day to enjoy my surroundings.
	____ I can easily spend time and money on myself.
	____ I have a place in my home for privacy and solitude.
	____ I have many friendships and make time with my friends a priority.
	____ I laugh many times a day and am always looking for ways to have fun and a good time.
	____ Total

SCORING ANALYSIS

A score of 7 or lower in any section indicates that this area of your life could be a source of energy drain. Choose energizing strategies that focus on any area that is an energy drain for you.

Karen Rowinsky

Now that you have an idea of what drains your energy, you are ready to start picking strategies. Start by choosing strategies in the area where you most need more energy. The more you enjoy a strategy, the quicker it becomes a habit, and you derive the most benefit. The operative word here is "fun!" One more thing before you get started. Even if you feel generally lethargic and depleted, most agree that there are times when you have more energy. Some of us are a "morning person" or a "night owl." Our downtimes during the day might be right after lunch or late afternoon. One key to maximize the energizing strategies: Figure out when you need them the most.

How? Keep an Energy Diary for four days, including weekdays and weekends. Use the form that follows as an example. Keep a copy handy for noting your energy level at each particular time. Or if it is more convenient, jot down how you feel in your daily planner or computer desktop. Check in on yourself throughout the day to assess your energy level at given intervals.

DAILY ENERGY DIARY

Complete this checklist for four days. Be sure to include weekdays and weekend days. If you are on a different schedule of waking or sleeping than those indicated, change the categories to reflect your schedule. At each time noted, assess your energy level. If you feel like you have more than average energy, put ↑ in the corresponding box. If you have less than average energy, put ↓ in the corresponding box. If you have average energy, use —.

	DAY ONE	DAY TWO	DAY THREE	DAY FOUR
Upon Waking up				
Breakfast				
Mid-Morning				
Lunch				
Mid-Afternoon				
Late Afternoon				
Dinner				
Mid-Evening				
Late Evening				

After the fourth day see if you notice any patterns in your daily energy level. When possible, arrange your calendar to make good use of your high-energy times. When you can't choose and have to do something at a low-energy time, find one of the 50 energizing strategies to give you that needed burst of energy.

Karen Rowinsky

Part Two:

Using Your Body

*M*any of us assess our energy level by tuning into the sensations in our body. When we are free of annoying aches and pains, we feel energetic, flexible and limber, and we experience strength in our muscles. So why don't we ensure that our body always works this way?

Does this scenario sound familiar? You know that it's important to make exercise a regular part of your life. Only 30 minutes of aerobic exercise four to five times per week goes a long way to make your heart healthy, and that exercise will give you more energy by raising your metabolism. You want to do it and so you start. One, two, even three weeks go by and you're exercising and beginning to feel good, maybe even a little smug—who said this was so hard? Then something happens: You have to meet with an important client during your regularly scheduled exercise time; you get a cold and don't feel like working out; you accompany your daughter on her class field trip instead of going to the gym.

You give in and before you know it, you've missed exercising on a regular basis. Pretty soon you're down to maybe twice a week. A few months of exercising only sporadically and you feel like it will take an incredible act of will to resume your regular exercise program. If this is you (it's most certainly me!), we can still energize our bodies when not exercising regularly. The following strategies will not only help get your body moving but will offer you other ways to use your body for increased energy.

Karen Rowinsky

1. Taking the Long Way Around

Without regular exercising, we need to get our bodies moving whenever and wherever. Take the long way around whenever possible. Instead of playing "Find the Closest Parking Space," park your car in the space farthest from the entrance. You know what I mean: Stop circling the mall parking lot. Make a promise to yourself that you will park as far away as you feel safe.

Okay, I will admit that I've been known to shop in one anchor store in the mall and then go out to my car (parked next to the entrance) and drive across the lot to the other anchor store to avoid walking the length of the mall. This is not helping me get my body moving. Make it a practice every time you go to the mall to take at least one brisk lap during your shopping. You're saying you don't have time but I'm talking brisk and you're actually getting errands done at the same time!

Energizing Tip #1:

Park in a (safe) parking space farthest from the entrance.

2. Doing the Aisles

*P*arking far away works at the grocery store or the hardware store too. Next time you need to run in for just a "few things," be sure to walk briskly up and down every aisle before making your way to the check-out. Caution: Don't try this weekdays, between 5 and 6 p.m., unless you want to incur the wrath of people in your way as you do your aisles.

Parking far away and then *Doing the Aisles* at the grocery store qualifies as exercise to me. Experts now say that even 10-15 minutes of exercise has benefits. Besides, who ever heard of a 10-minute trip to the grocery store?

Energizing Tip #2:

Be sure to walk briskly down every aisle in every store whenever you shop.

Karen Rowinsky

3. The No Parking Zone

*N*ow that you're home, don't leave the toilet paper and toothpaste you bought at the grocery store at the bottom of the steps. Don't wait for your next trip up to the bathroom—take it up right away! In fact, make the bottom of your steps a *"No Parking"* Zone.

If you don't have a second floor, this is also true for the basement. Every time you have something to go upstairs or downstairs, take it. If you have neither a second floor nor a basement, be sure to take more steps rather than save steps as you go about your household duties. You've just moved your body around!

Energizing Tip #3:

Never leave anything at the bottom of a flight of stairs.

4. Get Up and Get Going

*O*kay, so now it's evening and you're sitting in front of the TV. Don't even say it. I know you're thinking, "Who has time for TV?" But let's just say on the rare occasion that you do sit down for more than 15 minutes, be sure to get up and do something.

If you are watching TV, then whenever a commercial comes on, *get up and get going.* Go to the bathroom, change the laundry, make a phone call, get a glass of water, get a bag of chips and a soda…just kidding, I wanted see if you were paying attention!

Energizing rule: Every 15 minutes or so of couch time should be followed by 3 minutes of moving time. Call it the *15 to 3 Energizing Ratio.*

Use this strategy anytime you are sitting for long periods of time: Using the computer, reading, or even working at your desk. Apply the *15 to 3 Energizing Ratio* and you've just moved your body around!

Energizing Tip #4:

Get up off the couch every time a commercial comes on the television.

Karen Rowinsky

5. The 15 to 3 Ratio

*I*f your work does not require physical exertion, apply the *15 to 3 Energizing Ratio* at work too. It's easy: Don't save up your trips to the copy machine or printer until you've processed a morning's worth of letters. Get up and retrieve them every time you press "print."

I used to work in a hospital. Before I started using energizing strategies, I planned the excursions out of my department, trying to use my time and energy economically. Once I started using energizing strategies, the hospital became a wonderful place to get some exercise without taking time to change into sweats. I learned to get out there and walk those halls. Apply the *15 to 3 Energizing Ratio*: Volunteer to pick up things from other departments for your coworkers or help them out by taking their mail to the mail room.

Energizing Tip #5:

Have three minutes of moving around time for every fifteen minutes of downtime.

6. Take the Stairs

*I*f you work in a building with elevators, make a pact with yourself that you will never take the elevator one floor up or two floors down. Once you get used to this, you can increase to walking two flights up and three down. Pretty soon, you'll recognize that the other people in the stairwells are the ones with more energy (and more muscular calves!). Soon you'll be one of them and that is good.

Energizing Tip #6:

Never take the elevator one floor up or two floors down.

7. It's Time for Recess

I don't relish exercise. In fact, I've never met an exercise I really liked. But that doesn't mean that I can get away without doing some. I play mind games with myself in order to exercise. This might work for you too.

Instead of working out, I have *Recess!* Do you remember in elementary school those 15 minutes in the morning and afternoon when you ran around the playground, stopped for a quick game of tag, climbed up and over a jungle gym, or played a mean game of tetherball? You were assured 15 minutes of exercise twice a day.

So what's keeping us from having *Recess* as adults? Instead of your coffee break, do a quick walk around the block (or the halls if the weather is inclement). Grab a friend and spend lunch at the bowling alley.

At home, challenge your kids to a quick game of "horse" or take your bike for a quick spin around the block before dinner.

Choose something that gets your body moving but doesn't require a change of clothes, much preparation, equipment, or even sweat. Don't think that you have to have at least an hour. Less is okay. Think *Recess!* The 15 minutes you spend building energy will be well worth it.

Energizing Tip #7:

Instead of a coffee break, take recess by doing a fun physical activity.

8. The Nose Knows

*I*sn't it amazing? The instant you smell a particular fragrance you are immediately transported to a time when you smelled it in the past. The olfactory system (our sense of smell) has an incredible memory. Real estate agents have figured this out. That is why they recommend that home sellers bake cookies or bread or simmer some vanilla extract and water on the range before showing their home to prospective buyers. Those aromas immediately signify feelings of hominess and comfort to many people.

We can use this power to give us more energy. Think about the time in your life when you felt most energized and recall a smell that reminds you of that time. Perhaps you were actively involved in sports, it might be the smell of Ben-Gay. Or maybe it was around the time when you had a baby. Most people are exhausted when they become new parents, but the feelings of delight and excitement a new baby brings actually energize them. If this kind of memory does it for you, then maybe the fragrance of baby lotion will be one that triggers your brain into experiencing those energized, vital feelings again.

For me, the time in my life when I was most energized was in high school. I was a perky, bubbly, boy-crazy girl with a bounce to my step. Boys then wore one of two colognes—English Leather or Jade East. I preferred the English Leather guys. When I was in the vicinity of a boy drenched in this fragrance, my heart would beat faster; I would get almost tingly inside.

That "boy smell" still gets me going today. When I realized how powerful this fragrance was for me then, I decided to see if it still was available. It is! When I really get draggy or need an instant boost, I open up that bottle for just a little sniff and

I start to tingle like that boy-crazy high school girl I was many years ago.

What kinds of fragrances bring back your good memories, when you felt zesty and full of energy? Once you decide, stock up on samples of these fragrances and pull them out whenever you want to tingle.

Energizing Tip #8:

Find an energizing fragrance and take a whiff when you need a lift.

9. Feeling Juicy

*D*o you drink 8-10 eight-ounce glasses of water each and every day? Water is the most vital nutrient for maintaining good health but few of us think of water when we need an energy boost. When our body is properly hydrated, it functions better, working more efficiently and comfortably. You've heard the saying, "works like a well-oiled machine." When we drink enough water, our body does.

Normally, I didn't drink a lot of water. Often from meal to meal not so much as a sip of water passed my lips. When researching energizing strategies, I learned the importance of drinking water. Most of us walk around dehydrated almost every day, and in fact, by the time we become aware of feeling thirsty, we are actually well on our way to dehydration.

I decided to experiment to see if just by drinking water I would feel more energy. After drinking the minimum requirement for about three weeks, I had more energy! My body felt different. It seemed to feel more comfortable. I felt I moved with more ease and it took less effort. My skin looked better, not dull, and it seemed to glow. I actually felt juicy! Juicy is a good feeling too. When we feel juicy, we feel more alive.

If you are not a water drinker or stopped drinking enough water lately, try the following strategies to increase your water intake. Drink your eight glasses of water each day for three to four weeks, and I'm sure you will never allow yourself get dehydrated again.

- Build your water intake gradually adding two glasses a day for the first week. The following week, add two more until you are up to your eight glasses a day.

- Drink two glasses early in the morning, two more by noon, two before dinner, one with dinner and one before bedtime.

- Use small containers for your water so the amount doesn't seem overwhelming. An eight-ounce glass of water is just one cup—smaller than most drinking glasses.

- Treat yourself to bottled water if it tastes better to you. It's more convenient and it's easy to get into the habit of never leaving home without a bottle in tow. Use the pint or liter size and you only have to drink four bottles a day! If you're worried about the cost, refill each bottle at the tap or drinking fountain a few times before you discard the bottle.

- During hot weather, keep plastic bottles of water in the freezer. Leave the bottle in the car when you're out and about. It will give you a ready supply of cool water as it defrosts. Don't drink the water if the bottle and water become hot and don't try this with glass bottles!

Coffee, tea, soft drinks, and milk are not substitutes for water. Drinks containing caffeine actually draw the water from our system. If you must have them, use these fluids in addition to your minimum daily water requirements.

The only downside to drinking a lot of water each day is that you'll be going to the bathroom more. But hey, your trips to the bathroom count for keeping your body moving!

Energizing Tip #9:

Take a bottle or travel mug of water with you every time you get in your car.

10. Are We What We Eat?

*W*hen it comes to energy, we are indeed what we eat. By the time we reach adulthood, we know that if we eat a diet low in fat and moderate in carbohydrates we would be healthier, our weight would be appropriate for our height and frame, and we would definitely have more energy. We would feel better, look better, and not cringe at even the thought of clothes shopping. We know all this like we know we have to breathe. Still let's face it, most of us at some time or another do not have good eating habits, let alone maintain a comfortable weight.

A diet low in fat energizes us because our body uses quite a bit of energy digesting the fat we eat. You can use this information as an energizing strategy. The next time you anticipate needing either physical or mental energy, try not to eat a meal or snack high in fat two hours or so before. For example, if you have an afternoon meeting requiring a great deal of mental effort, choose a chef's salad with just a little dressing rather than a burger and fries for lunch. Now you can use your energy efficiently on the important meeting rather than on digesting French fries.

Speaking of salads, here's a quick tip. To avoid the flavor of low fat or no fat dressings, have your favorite dressing "on the side." Then, dip each forkful of salad very sparingly into the dressing. With just the tiniest amount of dressing on your fork full of salad, your tongue tastes the dressing first. It's as if your salad is covered in dressing. Try it! You'll finish all the salad on your plate before you've even put a dent in the salad dressing.

Okay, back to eating for energy. Most of us, when we think of eating something to give us energy, will automatically grab a candy bar or anything high in sugar. Ingesting sugar does give us an immediate burst of energy but the problem comes after that initial burst. We take a dive. Our energy level shoots up with sugar but that feeling of energy is almost immediately replaced by feelings of lethargy.

So next time you need a quick energy fix, eat an apple, pear, or a handful of raisins. These fruits not only have natural energizing sugars, but they are high in boron. Boron is a great boost as it increases our mental alertness and clarity.

Energizing Tip #10:

Eat an apple, pear, or raisins when you need some energy.

11. Make Time to Let Go

---

*O*ur body holds tension in certain sets of muscles; sometimes in several places around the body. When our muscles are tense, we are contracting them. When we contract a muscle, we are wasting energy that could have been put to better use.

Think about it. Where do you hold your tension?

- *Around your eyes?* Is your brow usually furrowed? Do you find yourself squinting even when you're not outside in the sunlight?

- *In your mouth and jaw?* Does your tongue have teeth marks down either side? Is your jaw constantly clenched? Do you find it hard to consciously relax your jaw and tongue?

- *In your neck and shoulders?* Does your neck usually feel tight and stiff? Does it feel like you are stretching your neck when you turn your head from side to side? Do you hold your shoulders in a relaxed position or are they hunched? Are your shoulder blades squeezed together instead of in the normal relaxed position?

- *Down your back?* Do you suffer from chronic back pain and therefore tense your muscles to guard against the pain? Do you find your hand frequently reaching around to massage your back? Do you constantly ask your friends or family members to rub your back?

- *In your abdomen?* Our mothers taught us to hold in our stomachs but do you find that you do this not to look good but when you are feeling stressed? Do your abdominal muscles feel sore even when you haven't done your regular regimen of sit-ups?

Karen Rowinsky

- *In your arms or legs, hands or feet?* Do they ache at the end of the day? Do you notice the half moon marks of fingernails digging into the palm of your hand? Are your toes curled more often than not?

It's natural to hold tension in our muscles, but more so in today's stressful world. We are actually training our muscles to be tense. To save energy, we need to interrupt this vicious cycle. Once you figure out where you hold your tension, make a concerted effort to release the tension there periodically throughout the day and evening.

Establish some muscle-relaxing triggers. While you're driving, you might focus and then release your tense muscles whenever you come to a red light. (This is very helpful if driving makes you crazy and you want to avoid road rage!) Or use the telephone as a trigger. When it rings, relax your tense spots and then answer. Find things that you do repetitively during the day like drinking water or going to the bathroom. Use those times to prompt you to relax your muscles. Not only will you feel better (and look better) but, by not having those muscles in a constant state of contraction, you will have extra energy to do something that REALLY feels good!

Energizing Tip #11:

Find cues during your day to remind you to release contracted muscles.

12. S-t-r-e-t-c-h It Out

*T*his three-minute exercise is guaranteed to give you an energy boost. You don't have to be in great physical shape and you can add your own special touches to make it work best for you. Once you run through this exercise a few times, you will be able to do it in about two to three minutes. It helps at first to have someone read the steps to you while you are doing them.

- Stand up straight with your feet about 18 inches apart.

- Take a deep breath in through your nose while slowly counting to four and exhale through your mouth while counting to four again. Imagine filling your body with air and then slowing letting it out through your mouth.

- Raise one arm up toward the ceiling. Reach as high as you can, making the stretch in your arm muscles slow and easy—no jerky calisthenics here. Slowly lower your arm.

- Raise the other arm in the same fashion and then lower it.

- Raise both of your arms and while they are reaching towards the ceiling, stretch out your fingers—wiggle and stretch them until they feel comfortable.

Take another deep breath in through your nose and out through your mouth.

- Slowly raise one shoulder up toward your ear and then release. Do it with the other shoulder. Then raise them both at the same time. Release.

- Slowly rotate one shoulder in a circle, rolling forward and then around. Rotate the other shoulder. Then rotate both at the same time.

Karen Rowinsky

- Gently stretch your neck to allow your chin to rest on your chest. Hold it there for a few seconds, then slowly raise your head to the forward-looking position. Gently stretch your neck, allowing your head to fall toward one shoulder. Return to the upright position and then gently stretch, falling towards the other shoulder. Do not stretch your neck towards your back. Doing so may worsen any undiagnosed disc problems. Repeat the front and side stretches, always returning to the upright position. Don't just roll your head around on your neck because you can injure yourself if you do it that way.

Take another deep breath in through your nose and out through your mouth.

- (Don't do this part if you have bad knees or if it causes you pain in your knees.) While your arms are comfortably outstretched to either side, hold your back straight and gradually bend your knees. Go down as far as comfortable with your knees pointing in the same direction as your feet. Then, slowly move your body upwards by straightening out your knees. The object is a gentle stretch while not bending over at the waist. Take a second and see yourself as a graceful ballet dancer! Repeat one or two times.

- Keeping your feet about 18 inches apart, push your hips to one side. Slightly bend the knee on the side you are stretching towards while keeping the other knee unbent. Resume the straight-ahead position and then gently stretch at the hip towards the other side, bending the knee on that side. Stretch gently and slowly, once or twice on each side.

- Roll your hips around and tilt your pelvis as if you are doing a belly dance. Reverse directions and roll the other way.

- Lift one foot an inch or so above the floor and stretch your toes. Then repeat with the other foot.

Take another deep breath in through your nose and out through your mouth.

- (Don't do this if you have back problems or if it makes you dizzy.) Using your head and arms as a weight, gradually stretch your back by letting your arms and head drop slowly toward the floor. Stretch each vertebra out until they all get to a comfortable stretch. You don't have to touch your fingers to the floor. In fact, you might want to comfortably flex your knees. Dangle your arms for about 30 seconds. Slowly bring your body to an upright position stacking one vertebra on top of the other.

Take another deep breath in through your nose and out through your mouth.

The great thing about this exercise is that in two to three minutes you feel refreshed and revitalized. Do it several times during the day. Do it when you feel yourself slowing down or getting bored with something that must get done. Also do it when you get home from work. Before going into the house, take two minutes to stretch in the garage. It will give you the burst of energy you need for what you have to do when you arrive home.

Doing it to music is a real enhancement to this exercise. Find some privacy, put on a nice easy tune, and stretch and sway to the melody. You'll feel invigorated at the end of just one short song!

Energizing Tip #12:

Take frequent stretch breaks during the day.

Karen Rowinsky

13. Sit Up Straight

*O*kay, I know I'm not your mom, but in this case she was right! Body language can have a direct impact on energy level. Body language can be an outward expression of what is going on inside. It's the way we position ourselves physically. People take in our body language as well as our words when we communicate. We even react to our own body language, acting and feeling in a way that reflects it.

Think about it. Look at the way you are sitting as you are reading this. Most of us do not have good posture. Are you slumped in your chair, shoulders rounded, chin resting on your chest? Take a deep breath, exhale, and then sit up straight. Square your shoulders and hold the book in a way that allows your head to rest comfortably on your neck. Do you notice the difference? When we're tired, depressed, even stressed, we slump. It's as if we feel the weight of the world on our shoulders. Just the act of sitting up straight makes us feel more in control and can help us feel energized.

Poor posture is a bad habit. But it can be corrected. When we do certain activities for long periods of time we tend to develop poor posture. Working at a computer, studying, reading, doing needlework, watching television, or even driving a car can be conducive to poor posture.

Standing with slouched shoulders and a sagging belly makes a person appear depressed and incompetent. Standing that way can send the same message to our inner self. I can tell in an instant when a friend's self esteem is low or she's had a hard day just by seeing her walk toward me. Her head is bent down, her shoulders are hunched, and her gait is slower. Her posture mirrors how she is feeling about herself at the moment. No wonder we have the expression "chin up." I know my friend can start feeling better by lifting her chin and not slouching.

To check your posture, stand straight with your back against the wall and chin parallel to the floor. For correct posture, the back of your head, upper back, buttocks, and heels should touch the wall. There should be gentle inward curves at your neck and lower back and a gentle outward curve at your upper back. The same curves should be apparent when you sit.

Again, we have another example of how mom knew best. By sitting or standing up straight, you will feel better, look better, and feel energized. You'll also be sending the world, and yourself, the message that you are vital, competent, and alive!

Energizing Tip #13:

Have your work station evaluated to be sure it is ergonomically correct for you.

Karen Rowinsky

14. That's the Rub

*H*ave you ever been hunched over your computer for hours when somebody walks in, puts their hands on your shoulders, and gives you a minute or two of massage? Just thinking of it makes my shoulders and neck relax. Massage, while relaxing, can also be a great energizer. My one caveat is that the touch must come from someone you like. Also, if you're the kind of person who doesn't like much touching, this strategy is not for you!

At one of my presentations while describing touch as an energizer, an audience member related that in her office, she and coworkers frequently will call out, "I need a backrub!" She qualified this by saying that she worked in an all-woman office, which made backrubs a bit less problematic.

You don't have to rely on others to use touch as an energizer. If you've been working at a keyboard for a while or working with your hands, take frequent breaks for a quick hand massage. Use the thumb of one hand to massage the palm and fingers of the other and vice versa. It not only feels good but also gets the circulation going so tired hands feel less achy.

The same goes for your feet. If you're feeling drowsy, slip off your shoes and give yourself a vigorous foot massage. Messaging your feet can be done anywhere, but it's really great when you do it at home with some peppermint lotion to massage into those tired tootsies.

Energizing Tip #14:

Give yourself a quick foot massage when you need an energy boost.

15. Take Care of Those Tootsies

*I*t would seem obvious that sore or aching feet can be an energy drain. Yet most of us don't take care of our feet until there's a problem. Treating your feet well not only makes life more comfortable but can actually add a spring to your step!

Besides wearing shoes that fit well and are suited to your activities, pampering your feet can result in increased energy. Try some of the following treats for your feet:

- After a hard day at work, take a few minutes to sit on the edge of the bathtub. Fill the tub with several inches of cool water. Place your feet in the water and just relax. After a couple of minutes begin stretching your toes and swishing your feet around in the water. Follow this by a brisk rub with a soft towel and you'll be ready to face your evening duties.

- (Don't use this strategy if you are diabetic, as a podiatrist should provide your foot care.) Treat yourself to a professional pedicure. It might seem like an extravagance but you deserve it! While enjoying it, pay attention to how it is done. You can do the same for yourself at another time.

Energizing Tip #15:

Don't wear shoes that hurt.

Karen Rowinsky

16. Wear It's At

I know I've done it. I know my friends have done it. I bet you have too. You've put on a few extra pounds and you notice that your waistband is getting a little hard to button. You decide to nip this in the bud and begin a healthy eating plan. You do great for a few days but then you have a close encounter with some cheesecake. Oh well, you'll start your diet again tomorrow! But, by the time you get around to starting that diet, your jackets are feeling tight around the shoulders.

So now here you are, walking around with pants so tight around the waist that you feel uncomfortable and you're trying hard not to stretch for fear that you're jacket will tear right down the back seam. In your discomfort, you think about buying some larger clothes but you nix that idea right away because if you go up in size, you will never have the incentive to lose those extra pounds.

You are right: Tight, uncomfortable clothes are a good incentive to get back to healthy eating habits. But in the meantime, you're miserable, out of sorts, and drained from the physical discomfort of wearing clothes a size too small. I'm not telling you to stop trying to lose weight. I am suggesting that tight clothing is an annoyance that depletes energy. If you want to feel more energetic you need to lose the tight clothes!

There are plenty of other incentives to lose weight. When your clothes get so tight that you are uncomfortable wearing them, either buy a few items to use until you lose those extra pounds or purchase clothes that allow you to gain and lose a few pounds without much notice.

For example, you might choose pants or skirts with elastic waists or perhaps elastic panels in the back or sides. Jackets and blouses can be purchased in styles that are looser and more forgiving. Also, many clothes are available in fabrics that have some stretch to them. You will be surprised how liberating it feels to not constantly suck in your stomach muscles or to reach for something without fabric constraining you. Remember, "free" is a word that we used to describe how it feels to have energy. Free of tight clothing, you will have the necessary energy to feel free to do anything you want including staying on that diet.

Another way to use your clothing as an energizer is to choose items in colors that stimulate you. If you normally dress in blacks, dark blues, browns, or neutral colors, be sure to have a vividly colored item or two in your closet. Bright red, pink, orange, or yellow make us feel vibrant when looking at or wearing them. Even if you can't lose the black, accessorize with splashes of bright, delicious color. This works especially well if you have to work all day, then do something in the evening without going home in between. Adding a bright colored scarf or necktie can be just the thing to give you that psychological energy boost to help you through the evening.

Energizing Tip #16:

Use colorful clothes or accessories to set an energetic tone.

Karen Rowinsky

17. The Eyes Have It

I walked into a coworker's office one day and saw her staring out the window. Without turning around, she told me to have a seat; she would be done in a moment. A minute later she apologized for keeping me waiting while she looked out the window but she was in the middle of preparing for an important meeting.

"Oh really?" I asked, "Do you always prepare for meetings by staring out the window and daydreaming?"

"No," she replied, "but I'm feeling exhausted and this meeting is going to require some energy. Staring out the window for a few minutes usually energizes me, especially when I've been working at my computer for a long period of time."

My coworker was right on target. Our eyes do get tired. Reading, doing computer work, even dealing with the pollutants in the air all put a strain on our eyes. Straining and squinting use up vital energy. Here are some strategies you can use to energize yourself by taking care of your eyes. When they feel comfortable you will too!

- *Eye Exams:* Be sure you are not straining your eyes because your glasses or contacts are not the proper prescription. If you haven't seen your eye doctor recently, make an appointment for an eye examination. As we age, this becomes particularly important because certain diseases and conditions of the eye occur more frequently.

- *Reading Glasses:* As we age most of us require some kind of reading glasses. If that's the case with you, wear them! We strain our eyes and waste energy trying to read something that just won't come into focus no matter how hard we try. If you don't want to wear them around your neck, buy several inexpensive pairs at the drugstore and keep one in each room of your house, your purse or pocket, your desk, even in your car. Have them anywhere you might have to read or see something closely. You will have a lot more energy if you slip those glasses on when you start reading rather than waiting to see if you will be able to read by squinting and straining your eyes.

- *Cleaning:* If you do wear glasses or contacts, keep them clean. Have a small bottle of eyeglass cleaner and a soft cloth at your desk, in the console of your car, and on your bedside table. Clean your glasses frequently. When you strain through dirty or smudged lenses you are wasting energy. The same goes for contacts lenses. Rinse them when your vision becomes foggy or when you have been reading or doing computer work for an hour or more. Contacts become dry; often a quick rinse will make your eyes more comfortable and enable you to see better.

- *Soothe:* Keep a bottle of saline eye drops in your pocket or purse and on your desk. A drop or two in each eye can be a soothing bath for tired eyes.

- *Relax from strain:*

  ▶ Staring off into the distance can relax the muscles surrounding your eyes. If you don't have a window, just gaze away from what you are doing for a minute or two. You will return with your eyes relaxed and refreshed.

  ▶ Take both of your hands and cup them over your eyes so that light doesn't get in. Hold them there for a minute or two while closing your eyes. If you do it periodically during your day, resting your eyes like this can alleviate strain.

  ▶ Rest your eyes by taking a couple of minutes to lie down with an eye pillow covering your eyes. Eye pillows are usually made of satin or silky material and stuffed with lavender or another fragrant herb. They can be purchased in most stores that sell lotions and aromatherapy oils. You can also buy a gel-filled eye mask. The mask can be heated or cooled, depending upon your preference, and placed on your eyes for a few minutes to ease strain.

▶ If you are sensitive to light, be sure to wear sunglasses when you go outside, even on cloudy days. Squinting wastes energy.

Energizing Tip #17:

Gaze into the distance to relax tired eyes.

18. It's Time to Tingle

Many people describe a "tingly" sensation when they feel energized. You might want to use the following to initiate or imitate that tingly feeling. Fool your mind into thinking that you have more energy than you actually do!

- Massage some peppermint-scented lotion into your temples, across your forehead, behind your ears, or at the nape of your neck. Be careful not to get it in your eyes. You can purchase lotion specifically formulated for this purpose or you can go to a store that mixes lotions while you wait. Start with just a few drops of peppermint oil in a small bottle of lotion. Keep adding more peppermint oil until you reach the strength that makes your skin feel tingly but not uncomfortable.

- Buy a small bottle of peppermint essential oil and add some drops to tepid bath water for a quick 10-minute energizing soak.

- Purchase peppermint shampoo, hair conditioner, and bath gel to get your day off to an invigorating start.

- My personal favorite is peppermint-flavored breath spray, which can be purchased at a drug or grocery store. It's usually kept right near the toothbrushes and toothpaste. It also comes in other mint flavors and cinnamon but I believe that the peppermint works best. Spray a few spritzes into your mouth when you need a blast of energy. Keep some in your desk drawer and use it when you have to field a phone call that requires an extra bit of energy. Put the person on hold for a few seconds while you give yourself a couple of spritzes. By the time you come back to the phone, you will be tingling with the energy needed to answer the call.

Karen Rowinsky

Keep some peppermint breath spray in your car. If you are beginning to feel drowsy while driving, use a couple of spritzes to wake yourself up.

Note: The first ingredient in the spray is alcohol, so use it sparingly. Also, if you feel very drowsy, pull over well to the side of the road or into a parking lot until you can wake up enough to drive safely to your destination.

Energizing Tip #18:

Use peppermint breath spray to give yourself a wake-up call.

19. It's Snooze to Me

---

*I*t's hard to feel energized during the day when you don't sleep well at night. If you have trouble falling asleep or staying asleep, here are some ways you may improve your sleep:

- *Routine:* Develop a same-time routine for bedtime and waking, even on weekends. Occasionally varying the times won't hurt, but try to be as consistent as possible.

- *Caffeine:* Don't consume any caffeine for four to six hours before your usual bedtime.

- *Food:* Don't overeat or undereat in the evening. A stomach full of high-fat foods can interfere with sleep because they are difficult to digest. Likewise, an empty stomach can prevent deep sleep.

- *Medications:* Ask your doctor or pharmacist if any of your medications could be disrupting your sleep. (For example, some over-the-counter pain relievers have as much caffeine as two cups of coffee.)

- *Exercise:* Regular exercise encourages easier and deeper sleep—but not within two hours of bedtime.

- *Worry:* If you start to worry about things at "lights out," set aside a time to worry earlier in the evening. Take control. Choose when to focus on what's bothering you. Establish a time limit (perhaps five minutes) for doing this, set a timer if you have to, and then when your time is up force yourself to think of something else. Important: Distract yourself after the allotted time.

Karen Rowinsky

- *Disruptions:* If you still can't sleep or if you wake up during the night and can't go back to sleep, go into a different room. While there, read or watch television. When you begin to feel drowsy, go back to bed. Your subconscious should associate bed with sleep or sex, not with lying awake.

- *Environment:* Create a good sleep environment with bedroom temperature in the mid-60s. Darken the room by installing heavy draperies or light-blocking shades.

- *Medical Conditions:* Some medical conditions can disrupt your sleep. Anxiety and stress are the most common causes of insomnia and usually strike around 3 a.m. Allergies, asthma, bronchitis, emphysema, sleep apnea, heartburn, arthritis, and menopause might also interfere. Talk to your health care provider if you suspect one of these conditions is disturbing your sleep.

- *Bad Bed:* Your bed could be the culprit. Goldilocks was right: Sleeping on a bed that's too hard, too soft, or broken down is difficult. A bed that does not provide adequate comfort and support can contribute to or cause a sleep problem.

Nothing can start your day off better than a good night's sleep. To feel energized all day, put your energy into finding out how you can get one.

Energizing Tip #19:

Go to sleep and wake up at the same time every day, even on the weekends.

20. A Power Nap Is Where It's At

I used to be the kind of person who couldn't nap. I'd wake up groggy and out of sorts. The rest of the day I felt worse and had absolutely no energy following that deep sleep. Then I discovered "power napping."

When most people nap, they will sleep for 30 or 60 minutes. When you train yourself to "power nap," you only sleep for 15 or 20 minutes at the most. At first you might not even fall asleep within the allotted time. That's okay. Even a few minutes of downtime revitalizes you.

Plan ahead for a power nap. One of my friends keeps a pillow and blanket in her car. (It helps that her car has tinted windows.) When she is feeling groggy in the middle of the day, she takes a break, goes out to her car, crawls into the back seat, and takes a 15-minute snooze. A travel alarm clock wakes her.

When you are feeling tired, you aren't at your best. Upon arriving home from work, immediately take 15 to 20 minutes in a darkened bedroom for a quick nap. Even if you don't fall asleep, that time is a good transition from one part of your life to another. Your family will be more than happy to cooperate by waking you in 15 minutes.

Schedule time for power napping into your day. You will notice the energizing results almost immediately. If more employers provided facilities for such napping at the job site, we would have far more productive workers. Forget the 15 minutes drinking coffee. Go for a 15-minute power nap, a quick trip to the bathroom, a drink of cool, refreshing water, and you will be on your way to several more hours of energized activity.

Energizing Tip #20:

Take a 15-minute power nap when feeling drowsy.

Karen Rowinsky

21. Every Breath You Take

*M*ost of us rarely think about the act of breathing. As adults, we might take 20,000 breaths a day. Normal, balanced breathing supplies oxygen to the blood which nourishes cells throughout the body, then removes the carbon dioxide waste. Breathing properly and practicing deep breathing techniques promote physical and mental well being. Paying attention to breathing can also be an energizing technique.

Try it. Take a deep breath, slowly and deeply though your nose. Let your stomach expand fully on the breath in, then contract completely on the breath out. It helps to visualize the breathing process. Some people imagine taking cool, blue air in through their nostrils. They feel and see it as it travels through the lungs, filling up all the little sacs, passing through the walls of the sacs, coursing through the blood stream all the way down to their toes. When they exhale, they see that cool, blue air change colors as it carries out with it all the stress and toxins we don't need.

Feel, listen and visualize the breath moving in your body. Long, slow breathing is optimal. In the beginning, the exhale usually feels easier and longer than the inhale and should be emphasized. Do not take in too much air at the beginning of your inhale. Let the breath enter and exit the body evenly.

Because it is easy to get distracted, you might want to say a word or phrase to keep your attention on each refreshing inhale and each relaxing exhale. As you inhale, focus on the feeling you hope to achieve as a result of this cleansing breath. When you exhale, affirm to yourself how wonderful that feeling is.

The next time you are feeling draggy or sluggish, pause a minute to focus on a refreshing, invigorating, breath of air. If this energizing strategy works for you, you might want to explore biofeedback, yoga, or meditation. Each of these disciplines enables you to get to know your body better. When you know what to do and how to do it, getting energy is as easy as your next breath.

Energizing Tip #21:

Concentrate on breathing in energy for a few minutes when you need some.

Part Three:

Using Your Mind

*J*ust like we assess our energy level by tuning into the sensations in our body, we also use our mind as a reflection of our vitality. When we are thinking clearly, speaking articulately, and creatively solving our problems, we feel vital and alive. When we feel our mind is muddled, have a hard time communicating, or can't seem to find the answer we seek, we feel drained.

How you think can have an impact on your energy level. In fact, sometimes the way we think about things can be as energy depleting as running a marathon. We can be our own worst enemy by allowing ourselves to dwell on all kinds of unproductive thoughts. For example, we can waste countless hours and lots of energy going over things that we have said or done. We use an incredible amount of energy by avoiding our issues and challenges, trying to keep our minds off what is bothering us. And, we waste a lot of energy on the "what if's" of life. Most of the time, we have no way to forecast the future. Still, we spend countless hours pondering what might happen.

Learning how to control negative and nonproductive thoughts is one way to conserve energy. Stimulating our mind increases our energy. The following strategies will give you ideas on how you can do both to increase your energy.

22. Use It or Lose It

*W*hether you call it a "senior moment" or a "mind glitch," the truth is that as we get older our mind and thought processes are just not what they used to be. A friend of mine claims that for the past ten years she hasn't remembered the name of any new person she met. Another describes those frequent moments when the word is right on the tip of your tongue but for the life of you it just won't materialize. Still another says her memory has gotten so rusty lately that her kids take advantage of it, sometimes having her believing that she approved an expenditure when she can't even remember them asking about it!

Just as daily weight repetitions in the gym strengthen certain muscle groups, mental exercises strengthen and enhance thought functions over time. While not a quick energy fix, the following activities can increase your "brain fitness" and in turn your mental energy.

- When dining in a restaurant or at a friend's home, try to identify the ingredients in the dishes you are eating. Concentrate on the subtle flavorings of herbs and spices. Ask the waiter or your host to verify your perceptions.

- A fun way to exercise your mind is to take time to do crossword puzzles and brainteasers and to play games that use memory and thought like chess, bridge, or Trivial Pursuit.

- Try memorizing your shopping list before going to the grocery store. Take a written list with you so that after you have filled your cart, you can check to be sure you have everything!

Karen Rowinsky

- Buy a 100-piece jigsaw puzzle and practice fitting the pieces together as quickly as possible. Note the time it takes you to do it. Do it again a week later and compare the times. Your time should improve the more you do it.

- Each time you come to the end of a chapter in a book you are reading, imagine yourself summarizing it as briefly as possible to someone who has not read it. Do the same for the whole book when you finish it.

- Develop a new hobby, such as learning how to operate a computer, going on-line, woodworking, playing a musical instrument, or learning a foreign language. With age, the learning is a bit slower but it is still possible. The energy we put into it will reap results.

The important thing about exercising your mind is to do it daily. Use a wide variety of interesting, fun activities.

By exercising your mind and getting it in tiptop shape, you will not have to work as hard when you need to use it. You will waste less energy making extra trips to the store for things you forgot, feeling embarrassed because you can't remember someone's name, or trying to find that word that is just out of your reach. Think of all the things you can do with the energy your save!

Energizing Tip #22:

Keep a crossword puzzle in the bathroom for mind exercise breaks.

23. Forget About It!

As much as we would like to consider ourselves mature adults, able to handle our differences with people, sometimes people make us angry and there doesn't seem to be anything we can do about it. How many times have you said, "I'd love my job if it weren't for so-and-so?" Or what about, "If my husband would only grow up and act like an adult, our relationship would be just wonderful."

People frustrate us for different reasons. I'm sure if we were honest with ourselves, we'd admit we do the same to them. In some situations, you can talk reasonably and work out your differences. But at other times, you could communicate until you're blue in the face, and nothing would change. It doesn't feel good to carry anger and frustration within us. Most of the time, we think there is nothing we can do about it and that we have to live with the frustrations.

But in reality you have complete control over the situation. You can't always change things, but you can control how you think and feel about things. In other words you have a choice as to how stressed you will be, how long you will carry a grudge, and how much you allow others get to you. You have a choice as to how you will act, how you will react, and just how far you will go to make things better.

Will you need to quit your job if you can't find a way to deal with the behavior of a coworker? While that might be an option, if you love your job, why let anyone else's behavior affect whether you remain? If your husband acts in a way that drives you crazy and won't change, will you divorce him? Instead of going to such extremes, many times we can change how we react to things others do.

So what does this have to do with your energy level? A lot of energy is wasted when someone or something gets on our nerves, ticks us off, or makes us so angry that we feel as if we are going to explode. Finding a way to deal with this anger is definitely an energizing strategy. You will find a lot of books on anger management, some in this book's resource section. They will help you determine whether you are dealing with severe, chronic anger or daily irritations. The following strategies may be worth a try when in the normal course of the day you feel like you're going to scream.

Actually, screaming can help. Of course you should do it in private and definitely not at the object of your anger. While screaming at another individual is not the solution, shouting and stomping your feet in private can release some of the negative energy. The key to this strategy is to do it for a set length of time. That's right, go down to the basement, set a timer for a few minutes and make like a dog howling at the moon. When the timer goes off, wash your face with cold water, take a refreshing drink of water or juice, breathe some deep breaths, and go about your business.

Sometimes you may want to say things to the object of your anger but realize that doing so would only make the situation worse. An alternative is to write that person a note describing what makes you so angry. Be explicit and direct. Write until you begin to feel the anger subside. Sometimes the absurdity of the situation will become apparent in the process and you will even start to have fun with it. But most important: Destroy the note immediately upon finishing it! Shred it or burn it—just get rid of it and send your angry feelings with it. That's not to say you shouldn't try to have a conversation with the offending person, but conversations (or even letters or e-mail) in the heat of anger rarely solve anything.

If you know your stressing or worrying is not going anywhere, consider exercising your control and sending it somewhere else. Write down what is bothering you on a piece of paper. Then roll the piece of paper into a ball and throw it into a wastebasket. If you prefer, fold it into a paper airplane and sail it away.

You've heard of messages in a bottle? Well we don't want to be environmentally irresponsible, so how about taking a marker, writing some words symbolic of what is making you crazy on a smooth rock, and then tossing the rock into a nearby river or stream. Or buy a bottle of children's bubble soap. Imagine blowing your angry feelings through the bubble wand so they are enclosed in the bubbles you make. Watch the bubbles float away until they burst and disappear, taking your dark thoughts with them.

Once you send your troubles away, think and act as if they were gone. Only you can do this for yourself. By letting go, you will have the energy you need to do the things that bring you joy, instead of bringing you down.

Energizing Tip #23:

Write down all the angry feelings you have towards someone or something.

24. I Don't Want To

*D*oing things we don't want to do is a sure-fire energy zapper. Seldom does a day pass without someone asking us to do something we really don't want or have the time to do. Even though it's an inconvenience or something we don't care to do, we either are too nice to say no or for some silly reason feel obligated to say yes. Once we say yes to an unwanted task, like baking cookies for a church function or driving out of our way to pick up yet another child for soccer practice, we feel stuck. The effort required to do it increases. We waste a lot of our energy being angry at the person who asked. In addition we may be mad at ourselves for accepting.

There is a better way! A very wise woman named Maggie once taught me a simple but amazingly sensible and helpful lesson. According to Maggie, life is too short to waste time doing things we don't want to do, especially things we don't have to do. When asked to do something you don't want to do, just say, "I'm sorry I don't want to." "What!" you say, "I couldn't do that." Of course you can! It takes some courage but it really works.

The first time I tried this was when a friend called late one afternoon and invited me to dinner at her house that evening. It had been a hard day and, while I usually never turn down a dinner invitation, I simply didn't feel like doing one more thing. (I had actually fantasized all day about curling up in my flannel nightgown in front of the TV with a bowl of soup for supper.) So I very nicely responded "I really appreciate your inviting me and any other time I would come but tonight I just don't want to." Silence…"What?" she replied. I answered, "I just don't want to come to dinner."

At that my friend started laughing. In between giggles she blurted out that she really hadn't wanted to invite me but that she had made enough and knew how much I didn't like to cook. She said it was a shock to hear the "I don't want to," but she was relieved. As my friend, she wouldn't want me to do something I didn't want to do. She also wouldn't have liked it if I had come just to avoid appearing rude or hurting her feelings. We both decided that while this was new territory for us, it is important for us to be able to say, "I don't want to" to each other.

When you think about it, saying "I don't want to" to almost anyone but your boss shouldn't be that hard. Most of us do more than our share for the PTA, Cub Scouts, or our service club. We should reserve the right to say truthfully, "Thanks for asking but no." Of course, when you do say that to the next person who calls for you to work at the rummage sale (something you may hate to do), she will probably hang up abruptly, saying to herself, "How dare she?" But if she thinks about it for a moment, she'll soon be asking herself why she didn't say no when she was asked to make the phone calls (something she may hate to do!)

Saying "I don't want to" every once in a while doesn't mean that you are lazy or that you don't find it important to give of yourself. What it does show is that you know yourself, you take care of yourself, and you realize that no one can or should do everything. With that knowledge and with the permission to decline requests for your time or your cookies, you should have plenty of energy left for the things that are important to you.

Energizing Tip #24:

Say "I don't want to" when you don't want to do something and then don't do it.

25. The New Golden Rule

Nothing is more enlightening than watching a friend overdo. We all know her. She runs from dawn until she drops. If she's not the driver, she's arranging transportation with the skill of an air traffic controller. If she's not baking for the bake sale, she's baking for an elderly neighbor. If she's not running a kid to the doctor, she's running her mother-in-law to physical therapy. All this on top of working full-time, doing laundry, cooking (or at least going through the drive-thru), and, if she is married, trying to maintain a relationship with her husband.

So what do you say to her, especially when she is stressed most of the time? You probably tell her to stop before she drops! You tell her you care about her and you think she is doing too much. You tell her that her kids don't need that extra violin lesson a week, that her church can go a week or two without her making those phone calls, that her siblings, or even a paid helper, can get her dad to his eye doctor appointment. It all seems so clear to you! You wonder why she is adamant about not changing and are frustrated when she responds with a big fat "Yes, but..."

Okay, I know this will be hard, but now put yourself in your friend's place. Does your life mirror your friend's? No wonder you, she, and the countless women we all know feel drained at the end of the day.

Here's where the New Golden Rule comes in: Do unto yourself as you would want your best friend to do unto herself. You could call it being your own best friend. Tell yourself to STOP. Enough is enough. We don't have to do it all! Numerous books and articles tell about leading a balanced life, but most of us don't realize that, unless we cut some things out, we will never find time for ourselves. We will never have the energy to do what we really want to do. Energize yourself by being careful about your commitments.

If you are really good at doing too much for too many people, you need the Platinum Rule. This rule requires you to ask yourself when you're feeling particularly tired or stressed, *"Will somebody die if I don't do this?"* If the answer is no, then tell your daughter that the retailers at the mall will have to do without her visit today. Let your son be satisfied playing on the community team rather than the traveling team. More than once a week, make reservations instead of dinner. Tell your best friend about that new restaurant you wanted to try and then plan to meet her there.

Energizing Tip #25:

Do unto yourself as you would want your best friend to do unto herself.

Karen Rowinsky

26. Should I or Shouldn't I?

*A*long with wasting energy doing things we don't want to do, we also waste vital energy doing things we think we *should* do. Women especially hear themselves saying the word "should" many times a day. Whether you *should* be bringing a homemade dish to the potluck or you *should* handwrite that note rather than send an e-mail, we are bombarded by "shoulds" all day long. If we don't end up doing what we think we *should* do, we start feeling guilty. Guilt is a prime energy drainer, drawing down our batteries as much as leaving the lights on in our car will drain its batteries.

When using the word "should," it's important to ascertain where the idea that you should or shouldn't do something comes from. Try this simple exercise. I call it the *Should Filter*. For the next week, every time you hear the word "should" coming out of your mouth or rattling around in your brain, pause and examine where it came from. Who told you, or where is it written that that particular thing should be done that particular way.

Most of us learn our *shoulds* from our parents. In fact, our job as parents is teaching a child how we think life should be lived. Even the rebellious among us are good listeners and early on we incorporate the *shoulds* our parents taught us into the way we behave. Some *shoulds* are timeless, like you should look both ways before crossing the street or you should respect your elders. But other shoulds that we learned are not as relevant to us as they were to our parents.

For example, my parents grew up in the 1930s and 1940s, so when I was growing up in the 50s and 60s, I was learning *shoulds* from the 30s and 40s. My parents in turn had learned their *shoulds* from their parents who grew up at the beginning of the 20th century. So here I am in my 50s living at the beginning of the 21st century and I am listening to *shoulds* that came from a century ago.

My parents' lives were very different from mine. My father worked outside of the home and my mother took care of the household devoting much of her time to raising four kids. While she worked hard with fewer conveniences than we have now, she felt she should have a hearty meal on the table each night, that shirts should be ironed right out of the dryer, that thank-you notes should be written immediately upon receiving a gift or dining at a friend's house, and so on.

I have two children. I worked outside of the home along with working inside while they were growing up. I felt I should have served wonderful dinners nightly but, more times than I'd like to admit, we grabbed a burger between work and running to evening activities. Sometimes we sat in front of the TV munching on a bowl of cereal for supper because I was too tired to cook. I spent a lot of time dwelling on what I *should* have done for dinner. This time would be better spent enjoying my children and my time with them. I was operating on a *should* from the 50s, which didn't work in the 80s and 90s. As much as I would have liked to have idyllic, nutritious meals every night, realistically we were lucky if I could pull that off a couple of times a week.

Had I known then what I know now, I would have cut myself some slack and would have stopped wasting my energy feeling guilty. My energy would have been better spent figuring out how to keep nutritious snacks in the car, then tooling guilt-free through that drive-thru.

How many times do you say the word "should" during the day? With all the demands and pressures we face in today's world, we can't do it all. But we can make a conscious effort to update the way we do things to fit the times. For example, instead of spending a lot of time preparing potato salad for the potluck, have your supermarket's deli department fill your serving bowl with potato salad. They'll even cover it with plastic wrap. Rather than slapping the price sticker on it, have them stick it to your finger. When you go through the check-out, just run your finger by the scanner. When someone asks, "Who brought the delicious potato salad?" Answer proudly and with a smile, "ME!"

We can help each other alleviate passé *shoulds*. The next time you go to a baby shower, give the mom-to-be a special gift: Have all the guests agree that she shouldn't send you thank-you notes. A simple thank-you when she opens your gift will suffice. Most new moms have little enough time with their babies before returning to work or taking care of other children at home. It doesn't make sense for them to waste time and a diminishing supply of energy writing those notes. Clearly a *Should Filter* is in order here!

On other occasions after applying the *Should Filter*, you may determine that the *should* is legitimate. The difference is that you will choose where you want to spend your energy, not just unthinkingly spend it like your grandma did.

Energizing Tip #26:

When you hear yourself say "I should," ask yourself if there is a good reason WHY.

27. Clean Up Your Act

S ome of us are more organized than others. If you are a naturally organized person or the kind who thrives in chaos, then move to another strategy. But if you feel that it takes too much energy to get your daily life in order, then read on. You may be surprised how a little effort can reap some energizing rewards.

Take a moment and think about how much energy you have wasted in the last week looking for something you've misplaced—your car keys, sunglasses, or even some clothing. If you're a parent, you know how frustrating it is when your child can't find the library book she borrowed. When you join in the search, you can't help but say, "If you'd put things away where they belong, you'd know where they are." A lot of energy is wasted searching for lost things when all we have to do is make a habit of putting things in particular places (and then remembering where those places are!).

Being disorganized wastes a lot of energy. Like making an extra trip to the supermarket because the list didn't include that vital ingredient. Or finding ourselves double-booked because the calendar wasn't up to date. Just think of the fun things you could do with the time you save by not having to search or re-do.

Many of us make lists to keep ourselves organized. That is good. To-do lists keep us on task. But sometimes to-do lists can be a problem. We have so much to do that when we look down the list, we get tired before we get started. A key to making to-do lists is to limit the number of items on them. Try to keep yours to no more than five or six items for one day. If you have more, start a new list. This list can be entitled "Things to Do When I Get Done." Then put this second list away. Psychologically even a pile of short to-do lists can depress us.

Try this: Always put something at the top of each list that can be completed quickly. You'll feel energized when you cross something off. Just the act of crossing it off gives you the burst of energy you need to complete the next task.

There are plenty of books to aid you in getting organized and even professional organizers who come to your home or office to show you how you can streamline and make your life easier. Check the list at the back of this book for some resources. If you think the chaos of your life is draining you, it might be worth the investment.

Energizing Tip #27:

Never have more than five or six items on your to-do list.

28. Reframe Is the Name of the Game

*T*hinking negatively can weigh us down. Some people are naturally optimistic and look at things from a positive perspective. They usually view a problem as a challenge or adversity as an opportunity. Instead of being stumped, they consider finding a solution to a dilemma invigorating. They view a difference of opinion as the chance to have a scintillating discussion. They are enthused by facing issues head-on rather than running from them.

But many of us feel worn down by life. Our glass is half empty rather than half full. Sometimes we feel that we have been dealt a rotten hand in the game of life. Rather than seeing what we can learn from it, we gripe, mope, and complain about things instead of taking action and control.

Letting life get to us robs us of energy. We feel we don't have what it takes to face the day. I once had a coworker who responded to every good morning greeting with "What's so good about it?" Even if her life at the moment was difficult there still had to be something that was good about it. It was a new day, full of possibilities. That day could be the day that things got better. By responding in that way she was setting a negative tone for herself and everyone else around her.

Just the simple act of exchanging one word for another or looking at something from a different point of view can give us more energy. If you are naturally a negative thinker, try a month of forcing yourself to see the bright side. Correct yourself every time you use the word "problem." Change it to "challenge." Focus on the solution rather than how bad you feel when things don't go your way. Shut your mouth when you hear that first word of complaint coming out.

I'm not saying that we have to always embrace adversity, but try a month to see what it feels like to see your glass half full. Cheers!

Energizing Tip #28:

Call your problems "challenges" and then choose to confront them positively.

29. The Write Way

For many of us, when we feel depleted or face challenges, it seems as if we've always felt that way. But in reality, there are many days (or at least many hours) where we feel vital and full of life, vim, and vigor. Journaling can help put our life in perspective so we don't only remember when we were tired and grumpy.

Journaling doesn't have to mean keeping a diary with a blow-by-blow description of your day. You can write about your daily thoughts and experiences, or you can keep a record in your daily planner or a little notebook when you've had a particularly energetic time. Note how you feel physically as well as mentally. You might even mention why you think you are experiencing the energy. To really make this work, it helps to get into the habit of jotting down some notes right before bedtime. You can review the times in the day when you felt great and what you did with that wonderful feeling.

Then when you're feeling particularly lethargic, read some of your entries. You might notice a pattern. For example, on the energy-filled days you may be eating better, exercising more, spending more time with friends, or completing a long-term project. Knowing this you can do two things: Realize that you haven't felt this tired forever; and second, choose to repeat what you did on the day you felt more alive.

This kind of journaling can also be useful when you are having downtimes. Write how you feel when you seem listless or lifeless and why you think you are feeling that way. The next time you are feeling particularly energetic, read these remarks. You might find a clue as to what caused the drain on your energy. When your energy goes south again, you'll have the insight to nip it in the bud or do something differently to raise your energy level.

Journaling is a great way to gather information about thoughts and feelings. It can also serve as a creative outlet, an organizational tool, even a stress reducer. You might want to look at a resource on journaling at the back of this book.

Energizing Tip #29:

Keep notes on how you feel when you have lots of energy.

Part Four:

Using Your Spirit

*O*ur energy level can be related to how we experience our body and our mind and it directly relates to how we feel about our life in general. When we feel sad, stressed, or even bored, our energy level feels as low as our mood. Yet when we feel happy, cared for, and satisfied we feel effervescent and have a spring to our step. Our spirit is reflected by the smile on our face and the twinkle in our eyes.

Using your spirit brings energy to your life. You may want to develop a strong spiritual self. Spiritual beliefs and rituals energize many of us. If you haven't paid attention to this part of yourself lately, now may be the time to begin a spiritual exploration. Living spiritually brings richness to our life. Prayers and meditations can be done at any time and in any place. Taking a few minutes for inner reflection can give you the lift you need.

The spirit within you may also be described as your "life force." It is that part of you which experiences the fullness of life and the joy that living holds. The following strategies build energy by increasing that joy and the pleasure you take from everyday living. Enjoy!

30. Give Us a Smile

Smiling is energizing. Not only does it exercise and stretch your facial muscles, and thereby generate energy, it is difficult to smile and still feel glum or lethargic. When you have a smile on your face, it's contagious. People react to you more positively. It's hard to be with a person who is smiling without doing so yourself. Have you ever watched someone get his or her photograph taken? Even when watching someone smile in that situation, we find ourselves grinning right back.

Did you know that your voice changes when you are smiling so that you can actually hear a smile? If you listen carefully to radio announcers, you can tell when they are smiling. So not only will your smile energize you, it can energize the person you're with, even if it's over the telephone.

Do you smile easily? Take a few days to notice how many times you smile during the day. A little Mona Lisa-like curve of your lips counts as much as a big toothy grin. The important thing is whether you are smiling often. If not, as silly as it may seem, try smiling more. At first it might feel forced (and it is) but eventually it will become a habit. When you wear a smile on your face, your whole demeanor changes. It's as if you are smiling on the inside, too.

Energizing Tip #30:

Check your facial expression during the day. If you're not smiling, say cheese!

Karen Rowinsky

31. Just Imagine

*J*ust imagine having all the energy you want or need. You can use the exercise at the beginning of the book not only as an incentive to use energizing strategies, but as a strategy itself. Your mind and body are connected. Imagine being energized, awake, and alert and when your mind experiences a feeling of being energized, your body can feel the sensation, too.

Here's an exercise to understand what I mean about the mind-body connection. Close your eyes and picture yourself in your kitchen. Imagine that you are standing at your kitchen counter. In front of you are a cutting board, a knife, and a bright yellow lemon. Look at the lemon and see its shape. See the shine of its skin. Notice the texture of its skin, the creases and tiny indentations.

Now pick up the knife. Notice the weight of it in your hand. Feel the texture of the handle against your palm's skin. Place the knife's blade on the lemon's rind and firmly cut a wedge. You will feel the resistance of the skin at first until the sharp blade cuts through. Almost instantaneously you can feel and see the lemon oil spray and the juice of the lemon wet the blade of your knife and pool on the cutting board. The fragrance of the lemon wafts up to your nostrils and its distinctive aroma brings back memories of lemonade or iced tea and lazy summer days.

Still imagining, put the knife back down on the counter. With your fingers, grasp the newly cut wedge of lemon. Slowly bring the wedge up towards your mouth. The aroma gets stronger the closer the wedge of lemon gets to your lips. Then imagine your lips parting, your mouth opening. You hold the wedge of lemon to your open mouth and suck on it.

Okay, back to reality. Did you experience your mouth puckering up when you imagined taking that suck of the lemon wedge? Even now, can you feel the increased saliva in your mouth as a reaction to the lemon's sourness? That is the mind-body connection. Your mind imagined sucking a lemon and your mouth reacted as if the lemon was actually there.

You can use this mind-body connection as an energizing strategy by doing an exercise similar to that of sucking on the lemon. Only this time, imagine what it feels like to feel energized. Picture yourself at a time when you do have energy. Use your senses to feel the sensations in your muscles, your lungs, your heart, and your brain. See yourself running, jumping, swimming, dancing, thinking clearly—doing anything you do when you feel vital and strong. Experience the blood coursing through your veins. See the oxygen molecules feed your muscles. Feel their strength as they effortlessly propel you.

A visualization like this need take only a minute or two. Once you create it, you can recycle it whenever you need that feeling and it just isn't coming by itself. Just imagine what you can do with the energy that will result!

Energizing Tip #31:

Use your mind-body connection and imagine a time of energy in the past.

Karen Rowinsky

32. Accent on the Affirmative

*T*he dictionary describes an affirmation as an assertion of the truth or existence of something. Affirmations are a popular technique used by successful athletes, entertainers, and business people. In an affirmation, we are giving ourselves a positive message regarding our capabilities. The more our mind hears such positive statements, the more we take as truth the message they bear.

We can use affirmations to instill energy in general or when we need a spurt on the spot. Choose a statement of intent and speak it aloud. Here is a sampling of energizing affirmations:

> *I feel energized and alert.*
>
> *I am strong and vigorous.*
>
> *I choose to be healthy.*
>
> *I am up to the challenge.*
>
> *I appreciate the gift of my vitality.*
>
> *I delight in my vim and vigor.*
>
> *I can get the job done.*
>
> *I enjoy my active life.*
>
> *I know how to have a good time.*
>
> *I recognize my power to choose.*
>
> *I live enthusiastically.*

Because our brain experiences our affirmations literally, always use positive statements. Don't use words such as "I don't feel tired anymore" or "I am losing my lethargy." Your brain will hear "tired" and "lethargy" and while these statements are fact, they will give your brain mixed messages.

When speaking your affirmations, visualize the actions. The use of your imagination will give more "oomph" to your affirmations. When you speak your affirmations, see them, feel them, smell them, taste them, and live them. By using all of your senses, your affirmations are powerful beyond belief.

After creating some affirmations that are meaningful to you, write them on index cards and post them on your bulletin board or on your refrigerator. Put one on the bathroom mirror for mornings when you just can't seem to wake up. Use one as a screen saver on your computer.

While you may feel silly at first, try a few weeks of using an affirmation daily. Soon they will become habit and I bet you won't be able to go through a day without one.

Energizing Tip #32:

Use energizing affirmations to recharge your batteries during the day.

Karen Rowinsky

33. Stop to Smell the Roses

*L*ife can get so busy that we don't stop to look at the beauty which surrounds us. That includes beauty in nature and in the people in our lives. The next time you are in your car rushing to a meeting and in need of an energy boost, take a few minutes to drive through (or even by) a public park or garden.

Just a minute or two will work. Notice the trees. Depending upon the season, see their leaves or branches swaying with the breeze. Notice their color and texture. Look at the grass. See the brilliance of the green. Enjoy the fragrance of all the growing things. Look up at the beautiful blue sky. Just making these few observations will give you a refreshing few minutes to clear your mind and energize you for your next task.

If you can make the time, get out of your car for a little stroll or sit for a few minutes on a park bench. Watching children playing, squirrels scampering, or a dog and its owner playing Frisbee can put a smile in your heart and on your face.

If you've had a particularly exhausting day, prepare for the hubbub awaiting you at home by taking a five-minute detour through the countryside. If you live in a city, a park or suburban neighborhood will do. Noticing the fields, the woods and the sky can change your mood. Beauty is an energizer. We just need to stop, notice, and breathe it in once in a while.

Energizing Tip #33:

Commune with nature by making a detour through the countryside or a park.

34. Ready, Set, Indulge

I ndulging oneself often has negative connotations. For example, we may describe someone who indulges herself as being self-absorbed, spoiled, or selfish. Who would want to be called self-indulgent? I do! Indulging oneself is energizing. The dictionary tells us that to indulge is to yield to an inclination or desire. There is nothing wrong with that. Much of the time we are pulled in a multitude of directions with obligations and commitments. We yield to other people's desires. When do we do for ourselves? And what do we do when we do for ourselves?

What I'm suggesting is simple, can be inexpensive, and won't take too much time, but it will provide you much pleasure and satisfaction: Treat yourself well, with an emphasis on the "treat!" The time and money you spend will be worth it, not only to yourself but also to the people around you. We all feel, act, and think better when we feel nurtured, taken care of, even pampered. Who better to do this for us but us?

So what do I mean by "indulge yourself"? It means going for the Godiva instead of the Snickers (the difference in price is about 50 cents, the difference in pleasure—if you love chocolate, you know!). Or if you are a tea drinker, savor your tea in a lovely antique cup and saucer rather than Styrofoam or an old chipped mug. My friend Billie has a collection of beautiful teacups and indulges herself with a tea party each time she takes a break. You can too.

Why wait for someone to buy you flowers? Indulge yourself with some stems dressed up with baby's breath and greenery. The few dollars you spend will be worth the pleasure, not to mention the pride you will feel in knowing that you are treating yourself well. If you have friends who live far away,

Karen Rowinsky

indulge yourself with a full 30 minutes on the phone with them. With today's long-distance calling plans, this will probably cost you only $3. Just think of the laughs, dreams, and pleasure you will share as you energize each other.

Indulging yourself doesn't have to cost money. How about indulging yourself by giving yourself some time—time to think, time to play, time to just stare at the ceiling. This may be the hardest to do but it may give you the boost of energy you need. Start small: Give yourself 15 minutes a day to indulge. You will be amazed how energized you will feel.

When we actively seek to indulge ourselves, besides energizing ourselves, we are benefiting the people we live and work with. A happy, smiling, and relaxed person can change the mood of the people around them. Why shouldn't we be the happy ones? Don't you feel more energized when you feel happy? No one deserves to be indulged more than you!

Energizing Tip #34:

Give yourself 15 minutes a day to do only what you want to do.

35. A Garden Tour

*D*rive out of your way to a neighborhood known for its beautiful gardens. Get out of the car and walk a few blocks to admire the colors and the scents. Notice the different kinds of gardens: Some are wild and wonderful, others are trimmed and tidy. Don't let yourself feel guilty for not having such lovely flowers in your yard or your apartment windowsill.

Enjoy the fruits of another's labor. Breathe in, feast your eyes, and admire the work of Mother Nature and her gardeners. If you enjoy looking at beautiful flowers, in only 15 minutes you will be energized without even getting your hands dirty.

Energizing Tip #35:

Take a 15-minute walk through someone else's garden.

Karen Rowinsky

36. A Mid-Evening Night Cap

*I*n the middle of the evening, when there are still things to do before going to bed, go outside for a few minutes. Look up at the sky. Whether it's starry or cloudy, it's always beautiful. Breathe in the scent of the night air. Notice how different it is from day air. Listen to the night sounds. Feel the solitude, even if you hear noises from the street.

See if you can pick out some constellations or find a planet or two. Make a wish upon the first star you see. If it's raining, a few minutes under an umbrella (just you and the night), will recharge your batteries enough to finish the dishes, help your child with homework, or even fold that waiting laundry.

Energizing Tip #36:

Step outside in the mid-evening for a breath of night air.

37. Rise and Shine

A friend of mine is a morning person. Because it fits with her body's natural rhythms, she chooses this time to energize herself. She sets her alarm 15 minutes early. Instead of picking up or packing a lunch during that time, she indulges herself in the quiet peacefulness of her home before others awaken. She makes a cup of her favorite coffee and sits down to savor the newspaper in peace. Those 15 minutes of solitude energize her and give her the jumpstart she needs to welcome the beginning of her busy day.

Energizing Tip #37:

Get up before the family for a few minutes of peace and quiet.

Karen Rowinsky

38. You've Got a Friend

You've got a friend, or do you? Sometimes our lives get so busy that we don't make time for friendships. That's a big mistake! Friends are incredible energizers. They help us put our lives in a context. They remind us of things that are important to us. They are great for a good laugh and offer a shoulder for a good cry when needed. Choose friends who energize you and reciprocate by energizing them.

Try to make a "date" with a friend at least once a week. This doesn't have to be a face-to-face meeting, although that would be wonderful, but at least make time to connect. E-mail is good but the phone is better. Don't feel like you have to have a long conversation; even five minutes can be a pick-me-up. Plan ahead and tell your friends what they do to energize you. Then they will know how to help when you are feeling lethargic.

Depending upon where you are in your life and how filled it is with work and family commitments, plan to spend at least one whole day with a friend at least twice a year. Better yet, a weekend getaway with a friend or friends can leave you refreshed and rejuvenated.

I can hear your "yes, but" as you read this. I know a weekend away may sound impossible, but the choice is yours. Try it once and, believe me, it will be so fantastic that you'll do it again. It doesn't have to be expensive either.

My friends Mary and Jeanie and I once took a road trip through Iowa. We left on a Friday afternoon after work. We decided that we would do all our driving on back roads instead of interstate highways. We stayed at inexpensive motels and ate cheaply, only splurging on one special meal. We laughed and talked and even had the luxury of time to be quiet with each other. We stopped whenever something caught our eye and had a couple of adventures, too. We were back by Sunday afternoon, our families survived, and we felt the effects of this time for months following. Photos and a video documented our fun. Even though that weekend happened many years ago, I can still look at those reminders and feel the excitement, pleasure, and vitality of it.

When you can't be with your friends on a regular basis due to your schedules or distance, you can still experience the energizing qualities of your relationships. Place photos of your friends on your refrigerator, your bathroom counter, or your desk. Keep photos of your friends at work, too. When you need a burst of energy, cast your eyes on the smiling face of your friend, remember a time you were together having fun, and you will soon feel that much-needed boost.

Energizing Tip #38:

Place pictures of your friends where you can see them during the day.

Karen Rowinsky

39. Love the One You're With

*I*f you've ever experienced infatuation or first love, you know what an energizer that can be. Talk about tingly feelings! You can't sleep, you can't eat, yet you don't feel tired. You are constantly ready to spend time with the object of your affection. Often those feelings of infatuation pass, even if we are lucky enough to have them signal the beginning of a long-term relationship. But who's to say you can't get them back? There are many rewards for trying; not the least of these is the feeling of more energy.

An easy and fun energizing strategy is to rekindle the romance of whatever relationship you are in. It takes some effort, but just remembering how great it felt should be incentive enough. Sometimes we get lazy in our relationships and the doldrums set in. If you want more energy, this might be the time to work your way out of Dullsville and into Wowsville. That means acting like you did when you were first wooing each other. You were probably nicer to each other, took better care of your appearance, and showed a real interest in each other's day and thoughts. In other words, you were on your best behavior!

If you are lucky enough to be in a committed relationship now, you might think about using sex as an energizing strategy. Please don't read on if you will be offended. Most people who are having a satisfying and loving sexual relationship feel they are happier and feel better about themselves and the world.

Improving your sexual relationship can be a wonderful energizing strategy. Hopefully your partner will want to cooperate. Make a pact to work on this. Should you call it work? Yes! It takes creativity, a time commitment, and desire to warm up a sex life that has cooled down. But the rewards will be more than worth it. Check out the resource section for books that might help. That strange thumping you hear will be the pitter-patter of your heart. That adrenaline you feel can be put to lots of good use!

Energizing Tip #39:

Make a "first date" with the one you love to begin rekindling the romance.

Karen Rowinsky

40. Are We Having Fun Yet?

Several years ago, someone asked me what I did in my spare time. I laughed saying, "What spare time?" The person pursued me, insisting that there were times in my busy day when I was free. I thought about it and realized that whenever those times occurred, I ended up doing errands. Yikes! Is that pathetic or what? So I vowed that no matter how busy I was, I would find some time to have fun every day, or at least every week. I was amazed at the results. Even a half hour of pure recreation refreshed and renewed me and left me feeling more energetic.

What do you do for fun? Do you have a hobby? Participate in a sport? Have a social life? Go to the movies? Shop? If you want to put a spring in your step and a smile on your face, you must have some fun. Build fun activities into your life and choose to do them when you need energy. The key is to find time for recreation in your life. If you have some spare time, make yourself do something fun rather than something you have to do. Treat spare time as a bonus and have some fun activities in mind whenever you get some time! You'll feel energized and ready to do what you *have* to do *after* having some fun!

Energizing Tip #40:

Find something fun to do and do it on a regular basis.

41. A Room of Your Own

*E*veryone needs some alone time—time when we can experience the peace of solitude and the pleasure of our own company. But often, if we are raising a family, going to work, or in a relationship, we may go days without one private moment. Having a place of your own and a few moments in it everyday can give you more energy than you'd expect.

A place of your own needn't be a whole room, although that would be great. A corner of your bedroom or basement will do. The key is to make it your own. Decorate it with things you like in colors that are pleasing to you. You need a comfortable place to sit, perhaps a reading lamp, a small table to put some photos and mementos on, maybe some candles, and a radio or portable stereo for music. Make the ambiance pleasing to your eye and your spirit. Then find time to use it!

Spend a few minutes there in the morning while everyone is still sleeping or when returning home from work. Be sure to schedule in 15 minutes or so in your special place between doing errands and work around the house. Escape there whenever you need a moment of peace or an energy boost.

At one of my presentations, a young woman said that with her two young children at home, she had no time or place to be by herself. I asked her whether she went to the bathroom periodically during the day. She replied yes and that her children even accompanied her there. What is wrong with this picture? What are we teaching our children when we allow them to take away the tiniest bit of privacy and alone time that we have during the day?

This young mother's children were three and five years of age. They were old enough to occupy themselves somewhere else when Mommy goes to the bathroom. She then said that if she shut the bathroom door, they just sit right outside of it, either talking to her or crying, depending upon their mood. What's more, when her husband is home, he's usually there right outside the door too!

Well, here is a new use for duct tape! If you have children or adults who won't even let you have a few minutes in the bathroom alone, place a small piece of duct tape on the floor about 10 feet away from the bathroom door. That 10 feet is your buffer zone. Tell the kids and whomever else that when you are in the bathroom they must stand behind that line. I know it sounds silly but, after a little fussing on their part, you will have the precious few minutes of privacy you deserve. You might even want to have a box filled with special toys and activities that you can bring out when it is time for your alone time. The important thing is that you not respond to their questions or fussing when you are behind your closed door (unless, of course, there is a possibility that they have gotten themselves into a dangerous situation).

If the bathroom is the only place you have to be alone, you can make it a special hideaway too. Bring in the candles, the music, and fill a basket with magazines or catalogs. You don't even have to pull down your pants. Just sit on the toilet with the lid down and delight in your few minutes of solitude and privacy. When you open that door, you will walk out a new woman—refreshed, renewed, and ready to be Mommy (or whoever) again!

Energizing Tip #41:

Make a place of your own in your home.

42. It's Kids Play

Kids seem to have boundless energy. They play and run and jump all day and still go kicking and screaming to bed. We can take a lesson from them and energize ourselves by doing kid-like things. It helps if you have the attitude that increased energy is more important than what people think about you.

Start a toy collection for yourself. Fill a box for home and for work with toys and playthings that are fun and goofy. Get creative. Your box can contain a ball and jacks, a bottle of bubble soap and a bubble wand; crayons and a coloring book; a slinky, a yoyo, or one of those paddles with the small ball attached by a rubber band; a kaleidoscope, a rubber ball to bounce, a funny puppet, and maybe even a jump rope. A trip to a toy store should give you lots of ideas. When you need a little more energy, pull out your box and play.

Depending on what makes you the most comfortable, you can either do this in private or ask your coworkers to join in the fun. A few minutes blowing bubbles, putting on a puppet show, or skipping rope will take you back to your childhood, make you feel like a nut, bring a smile to your face, and give you the energy you need long after you've put away your playthings.

When you think about kids, a lot of times puppies and kittens come to mind. If it's been a particularly hard day and you have lots to do in the evening, take a few minutes on the way home to stop at a pet store. Sounds silly, but think how cute it is to watch puppies cavorting with each other or kittens wrestling. The key is to leave the store without a puppy or kitten! Just enjoy them there because, I guarantee you, taking one home will only zap your energy.

Karen Rowinsky

What about the real thing? If you don't have children in your life, you might want to borrow one for a couple of hours a week. They are fun to be around, amusing, put things in perspective, and set a good example on ways to have fun in life. I'm sure that you will have no problem finding a child or two among your family or friends who could use some time playing with you (or whose parents could use a little downtime). If you don't know any, consider volunteering in a church nursery or at a day care center. If this strategy appeals to you, explore Big Brothers and Big Sisters. There are many children who are starving for adult company. It could be a win-win for both of you.

Energizing Tip #42:

Borrow a child to help remind you how to play.

43. Dance to the Music

Whether it's classical or rock n' roll, blues or bluegrass, jazz or just the tunes of your youth, music can set a tone, change a mood, even take you on a time-traveling trip. It is powerful and accessible and a wonderful energizing tool.

Earlier in this book, I mentioned that the last time I felt like I had all the energy I needed was when I was in high school. So it makes sense that the music of that time of my life would remind me of how I felt back then. I don't think I can listen to the sounds of The Supremes, The Temptations, or The Four Tops, without my heart beating faster, my body starting to move to the rhythm, and my soul being transported to the 60s. I am instantly that 16-year-old girl, full of life, exuberance, and promise. I had no responsibilities to speak of and the weight of the world was on my parents' shoulders, not mine. When I hear those songs, I'm back there. Before I know it, I'm energized and ready to dance through anything.

Use the music from the time in your life when you were most full of vim and vigor to spice up your life when you need it most. Build a music collection to use when you need to get yourself going. It's fun to make a tape with a mix of songs special to you.

Any other kind of lively music will work too. Tune in to a radio station with rock n' roll music when you're cleaning the house. Fold laundry to a rousing Sousa march. Play a tape of vibrant classical music on the way to work. Use lively music on a Walkman when taking a walk or doing yard work. Use music any time you need a boost. Have it ready and available so all you have to do is push a button to turn yourself on.

The lyrics can also energize. Find songs that give you the message you need to hear—then sing along and really let the words sink in. There are plenty of inspirational songs—some religious, some popular music. You can find inspiration in Broadway show tunes. I bet if you belt out a few verses of the "Impossible Dream" before doing something particularly daunting, you can't help but get it done!

Energizing Tip #43:

Make a dance tape of your favorite music and put it on for a quick dance and energy lift.

44. By the Book

*M*ovies and books easily transport us to another time and another place. In an instant, we are far away from our present-day cares and worries. While movies require a time commitment, books allow us to take short trips from our reality when longer adventures aren't possible.

Using books or magazines to energize is easy. While nonfiction works for some, for me, there is nothing like a few pages engrossed in an historical novel or a gossipy magazine to get my mind off what is dragging me down. The key to this strategy is the time commitment. I'm talking a few pages here, not an afternoon curled up on the couch with a good book (although if time allows, there is nothing wrong with that).

Whatever you read should be amusing, entertaining, and so far from your own reality that when you finish you will feel like you've been somewhere else. It should not require you to think, analyze, or learn. I'm talking no earth-shattering insights, just mind candy. Also, it should not be depressing or scary. You could choose quality paperbacks for this, or a literary magazine, but for a real escape, I'd suggest mushy romances, exciting spy capers, historical adventures, or an entertainment-type magazine (*People* instead of *Better Homes and Gardens*—the latter will just make you feel tired thinking about all the projects you should do!).

Keep a book at work, in your car, and at home. If you carry a purse or briefcase, stick one in. You don't need to remember the plot line or even the characters' names, so you can have several books or magazines going at once. Then, when your mind stalls in the middle of a project, or you've arrived home and just can't face making a meal right away, pull out your reading material and take a few minutes for a vitality break.

Karen Rowinsky

It may sound weird but it works. Five minutes engrossed in whether virile Lance will ever realize that sensuous Sabrina is the right one for him takes you away from your world. When you return, you'll notice that you will feel refreshed and renewed.

The one problem with this strategy is that you have to exert good self-control. Sometimes the need to find out what happens with Lance and Sabrina keeps you reading more than a few minutes. This can be counterproductive because taking time you don't have can stress you, and you use precious energy making up for it.

Energizing Tip #44:

Keep an engrossing novel with you for a few minutes of escape.

45. Exercise Your Funny Bone

*L*aughter is energizing. It is also a great stress reliever. There are all kinds of laughs, from rich, deep belly laughs to giggles that just bubble up from your throat. There are little, joyful "tee-hees" and there are ones that come out of nowhere but leave you snorting and wheezing. My personal favorites are the ones where you laugh so hard that your eyes tear, you can't catch your breath, and you go running for the nearest bathroom.

Laughing is good for you. It's good physical exercise. When we laugh, we exercise our diaphragm, abdomen, and occasionally the muscles in our arms, legs, and back. And what about that relaxed feeling after a bout of laughter? We secrete endorphins when we laugh, which causes us to experience a sense of well-being.

Everybody's sense of humor is different. My husband Rick and I were recently watching a comedienne on television doing a routine about her dog. She was going into great detail about this dog doing its "doody." I don't know why, but this expression struck me as funny. I couldn't stop laughing. Tears were streaming down my face as I glanced over at Rick, who was sitting there staring at me as if I was nuts. He saw no humor in this at all. And it's not as if he's a sourpuss. He is constantly telling me jokes he thinks are funny and to which I can only groan. Each of us finds different things funny—we may even laugh at something one time and remain straight-faced at the same sort of thing another time.

While some may think the Three Stooges belong in the "Humor Hall of Fame," others lean towards the humor on sitcoms. Some of us enjoy puns, others jokes with intricate plots. Probably the easiest laughter comes from laughing at ourselves. I'm sure I'm

Karen Rowinsky

not the only one whose life is rich with ridiculous moments. One of my greatest pleasures and energizers is to giggle with friends about shared experiences.

Laughter is infectious. Even if you don't find something funny, it is hard to be with someone who is laughing without feeling your own lips twitch into a smile. This can be helpful when you're working with a group of people on a project and the energy starts to flag. Take a few minutes for a laugh break. Tell jokes, recount silly stories, or reminisce about the last time you were working on a project together and the funny things that happened. When you get back to work, you'll realize that the energy gained was worth the few minutes spent.

There are all kinds of ways to bring laughter into your life. Start a busy weekend of household chores by renting a comedy movie. Bookstores have shelves and shelves of humorous material. Purchase some and keep it at work and at home for a quick funny fix. The Internet is also a vast source for jokes. Bookmark humor sites that you enjoy and then take a quick trip to them for a mood and energy lift, when needed. By exercising your funny bone you will not only be healthier and happier, you will also have an instant energizing tool to use when you really need it.

Energizing Tip #45:

Develop a "things that make you laugh" list and refer to often for a quick giggle.

46. It's Time for a Vacation

*I*f you enjoy taking vacations, be sure to plan one that will refresh you, not zap your energy. So often, we get exhausted just getting ready. Once there, we do so many activities that, rather than relaxed, our vacation leaves us feeling frazzled. Plan at least a day or two at home before returning to work after a vacation. This will help you ease into real life and extend the relaxed feeling you gained from the vacation.

Try taking several weekend getaways for a change instead of vacations that last one or more weeks. No matter where you live or for how long, there are places to explore right in your own backyard. Plan the getaway just like you would a vacation. You can be frugal, extravagant, or anywhere in between. Pick a destination you can drive to in a few hours: Just far enough away for a change of scenery but not far enough to experience driving fatigue.

You might want to stay in a bed and breakfast or a country inn. The variety and costs are limitless. The Internet makes it easy to explore and see where you'll be staying before you arrive. If you like the great outdoors, camping might be just the thing to refresh you. The important thing about a weekend getaway is that it is different from life at home. Don't plan too much to do and build in plenty of downtime. Sitting by a lake and reading, wandering through the shops in a small town—anything that will take little effort but give you maximum pleasure.

Make your way home early enough on Sunday to not feel rushed getting ready for the coming week. These mini-vacations can be taken by air also. Most airlines have Internet specials that greatly reduce the cost of the ticket if you can be spontaneous. You might choose a weekend to go away and

Karen Rowinsky

then wait until that weekend's Internet special to pick what your destination will be.

Finally, you don't have to go anywhere to take a vacation. You can get a quick, on-the-spot burst of energy by taking a short vacation in your mind! If you need some instant energy, just close your eyes and remember what your last good vacation was all about. Visualize the sights, sounds, and smells—anything to take you back to that lovely time. Then stay there for a few minutes for a great energy boost. If you haven't had such a vacation, make one up! Use your imagination to have any vacation you choose. Two or three minutes in the place of your choice will do wonders for your disposition and your energy level. It might even give you some ideas for the next time you want to really get away!

Energizing Tip #46:

Take two to three minutes to remember a time on vacation when you were relaxed and happy.

47. Become a Collector

*J*ust looking at an object that holds great meaning can supply us with energy. The object can symbolize a wonderful
moment in your life. It can be a souvenir from a past vacation.
It might be a small gift from a special person.

Surround yourself with these objects on your desk, your bedside table, your bathroom counter, in the kitchen, the living
room, or even in your car. Just one glance at a meaningful
object can represent the difference between having so-so energy and feeling invigorated.

My friend Leslie and I once took a very special trip. We both
had young children and rarely had time for ourselves. We
were quite proud of ourselves, taking a few days, making our
way up the California coast from Los Angeles to San
Francisco. It was truly a remarkable experience for us. Not
only was it a lot of fun but the trip had a profound effect on
our friendship. When we got to San Francisco, we visited
Chinatown where I bought a little inexpensive silk pincushion. That pincushion sits on my desk to this day, more than 13
years after that memorable trip. Most days I don't notice it
among the papers and paraphernalia but on those days when
I really need a lift, I seek out that pincushion and in one
sweep of my eyes I am transported back to that wonderful day
so many years ago. I remember the pleasure of that special
time I had with my friend. It brings a smile to my face and
lightness to my heart and, in that one second, I feel the energy I need.

Your objects don't have to be purchased. I collect rocks, a quite
inexpensive hobby! Each rock has special meaning to me.
Along with being beautiful in its own way, each rock reminds
me of a time that I particularly enjoyed. One is from a trip to

Karen Rowinsky

the seashore; another came from a hike I took with my husband. I have rocks from trips and rocks from the yards of my friends who live far away. None of them have magical properties on their own but, when paired with a delightful memory, each rock becomes an instant energizer.

If this strategy appeals to you, you might want to avoid the mistake I made, however. When I first started collecting the rocks, each one was unique enough that I could remember its story. As my collection grew though, it became harder and harder to identify a specific rock. Therefore, I suggest that you label your rocks from the start. Using an indelible pen on the underside of the rock, write a trigger word to remind you of where you collected it. You could also give each rock a number and keep a corresponding record of each rock's story.

It is amazing how a simple rock paired with a powerful memory can spark your energy. You too can become a collector—of rocks, souvenirs, small art objects, anything that will remind you of a very special time or adventure.

Energizing Tip #47:

Place an object in a strategic place to remind you of something special it represents.

48. Go with the Flow

_W_e all are creative. Some of us are more talented than others, but each of us, if called upon, can express ourselves in a creative way. That act of creativity can be a wonderful energizer.

Think about the last time you were creative. It may have been that you were creatively solving a problem. You might have been writing a poem, short story, or essay. Or maybe you were drawing or painting. Needlework requires creativity. So does interior decorating and gardening. You may express yourself by building something or designing a new way to do something. Or you may play a musical instrument or sing by yourself or with a group.

When we are in the midst of being creative or totally absorbed in what we are doing, we find ourselves in the _flow experience_ described by Dr. Mihaly Csikszentmihalyi in his book _Finding Flow: The Psychology of Engagement With Everyday Life_. (See Resources in the back of this book.) When experiencing the _flow_, whether in work, conversation, or hobby, time is suspended or speeds up. Hours seem like minutes. Feeling serene, yet invigorated, we're confident that our skills can meet the challenge. We need no reward beyond what is happening in the moment.

After experiencing the _flow_, we feel happy, content, refreshed. After experiencing it, we want more! In order to use the _flow experience_ as an energizer, we have to put ourselves in situations that encourage the _flow_ to occur.

You may want to set the scene so that you can easily slip into a creative mode. This might be the time to set up that darkroom you've always wanted. Maybe get that old piano tuned

Karen Rowinsky

and resume the piano lessons you quit in third grade. There are many opportunities to take classes at a local community college, arts center, or recreation center. This might be the time that you learn how to throw a pot, tap a dance, build a bookcase, or join your church choir. To use the *flow experience*, find the artist within yourself and give in to that creative force as frequently as possible.

Energizing Tip #48:

Experience the flow frequently by finding a way to express yourself creatively.

49. Doctor, Doctor Give Me the News

*I*n reality, it is a challenge to feel energized even if our body is in a healthy state. While optimum health would be fantastic, one doesn't need it to feel good. On the other hand, many times we feel tired, weak, run down, or lethargic because there is something wrong with our body or mind.

As adults, we often neglect little nagging complaints until they grow into full-blown symptoms. You and I both know that old saying, "An ounce of prevention is worth a pound of cure." Well, when was the last time you had a visit with your health care provider? How long has it been since you had a complete physical? Is your cholesterol and blood pressure in the appropriate range? Are you on schedule with age-appropriate screening tests? If you want your body to serve you, you must service it. We take our car in for periodic check-ups and oil changes but often we neglect ourselves. If you are due for a check up…go to the doctor!

And while you're at it, do you see your dentist regularly? It's not unusual to develop infected gums, especially if you are not brushing and flossing frequently. It takes energy to fight any kind of infection, energy that could be put to more enjoyable uses. When was the last time you had your vision checked? Poor vision can cause headaches, which are draining in themselves. If we are not seeing clearly, we can't think clearly. When we squint, we contract the muscles around our eyes. Contracting muscles in this way wastes vital energy. At the other end of your body, if your feet are bothering you, go to a podiatrist. Tired, aching feet make us feel tired.

Karen Rowinsky

As we have discussed earlier your mental health has an effect on your energy level, too. While exhaustion, listlessness, and lethargy are symptoms of clinical depression, you don't have to be clinically depressed to have your mental state affect your energy state. Many of us have experienced times in our lives when we have felt anxious or confused. Family members' problems might affect us as much as our own. Talking to a good therapist can be your first step to regaining your energy and positive frame of mind.

Some people are prejudiced against going to a therapist. They believe the purpose of therapy is to lie on a couch and tell someone your deepest, darkest secrets. That is far from the truth. There are as many kinds of therapy as there are issues. Some therapies are feelings-based while others teach practical solutions. Some therapies are based on family systems, yet others focus on the individual.

Struggling alone can drain more energy than if you were to stay awake for seven days straight. Sometimes, just a few sessions talking with someone who can offer you insights into what is troubling you, are the key to revitalizing your life. Talk with your physician if you think that this might be something you would like to explore. He or she will help you find the right therapist for you.

Energizing Tip #49:

Make and keep an appointment for a physical.

50. Do Not Disturb

*W*ell here we are at the last energizing strategy. This one might be the most surprising of all. Don't laugh, but sometimes you just have give into the lethargy. This means that there will be times when you are simply too tired, too lazy, too unmotivated, too negative, or too exhausted to even try to fight those feelings. At those times, don't! When you feel this way, just pull the covers up over your head and go back to sleep.

At some point, we all need a "mental health day" when we just want to say, "I don't want to!" to the whole day. There's nothing wrong with saying that. Sometimes, a day in bed, on the couch, or in a lounge chair in the backyard is the only thing that will help. You deserve a day every once in a while where you act like a slug or a couch potato. So do it.

There are two important things to remember. 1. Feel proud of yourself when you realize that a day of rest is a solution, and 2. Make no excuse to yourself (or anyone else) when you take one. You will be so much better for it. Don't worry that this will become a habit. If you are the kind of person who does too much, and you are if you are reading a book about energizing strategies, then you are not the kind of person who will get stuck on the couch.

When you choose to take a mental health day, make it a good one. Don't get dressed, or if you do, put on your most comfortable outfit. Skip the shower or, if you can't live with yourself, at least don't wash and blow-dry your hair. Brush your teeth but forego the makeup. Let the answering machine pick up your calls. Turn off the ringer on your phone lest you be tempted. Don't turn on your computer. You can live a day without e-mail. (Well, maybe!) Eat only comfort foods like soup, mashed potatoes...and lots of chocolate. Watch your favorite video. Doze off with a juicy novel. Wake to read a few pages and then doze again.

You might have to so some advance planning to take one of these days. If you have young children, perhaps you can make a childcare trade with another parent. If you have older kids, send them to a friend after school to prolong your vegging-out time. If you're responsible for making dinner for a spouse or your kids, tell them that tonight you just don't have the strength to even call for the pizza delivery. Let them be resourceful and find the number themselves!

This is your day. It may not happen too often (though I think you deserve one at least every season), so make the best of it. Put up the "Do Not Disturb" sign and, I guarantee you, the wonderful memories of your day off will energize you for weeks to come!

Energizing Tip #50:

Put out the "Do Not Disturb" sign!

A Word About Follow-Through

*O*ld habits aren't easy to break and new habits are sometimes hard to establish. Incorporating energizing strategies into your life, even if fun, is still a new habit. As you choose strategies, don't do too many at once. If you try to, they will have the opposite effect and you will feel more depleted than when you started.

After about three weeks of using a couple of energizing strategies, you might want to add more. Do it gradually. Also, continue to reassess. If a strategy isn't providing you the results you want, try another. There are plenty to choose from. I'm sure you will find a selection that will work for you.

Acknowledging a goal and sharing it with another is one way to help reach that goal. I call it accountability! Most of us do better when we know someone else knows what we're working towards. It's even better when we have a pre-arranged time to share our progress. As you embark on this energizing adventure, it might help to take someone else along for the ride. It will make it more fun and you'll even have someone to share your newly found energy with. Bon voyage!

Karen Rowinsky

Resources

*C*ountless books are available to aid you in striving to live a healthy, more satisfying life. You might find the following books helpful as you continue to build more energy into your life:

Beckford, Ruth. *Still Groovin: Affirmations for Women in the Second Half of Life.* 2000. Sourcebooks Trade.

Bodger, Lorraine. *2001 Ways to Pamper Yourself.* 1999. Andrews & McMeel.

Carter, Betty. *Love, Honor and Negotiate: Making Your Marriage Work.* 1997. Pocket Books.

Charles, C. Leslie. *Why Is Everyone So Cranky? The Ten Trends That Are Making Us Angry and How We Can Find Peace of Mind Instead.* 1999. Hyperion.

Csikszentmihalyi, Mihaly. *Finding Flow: The Psychology of Engagement With Everyday Life.* 1998. Basic Books.

Goodman, Ellen and O'Brien, Patricia. *I Know Just What You Mean: The Power of Friendship in Women's Lives.* 2000. Simon & Schuster Trade.

Gray, John. *Mars and Venus in the Bedroom: A Guide to Lasting Romance and Passion.* 1997. HarperCollins.

Hemphill, Barbara. *Taming the Paper Tiger at Home.* 1998. Kiplinger Books.

Jacobs, Ruth Harriet. *Be an Outrageous Older Woman.* 1997. Harperperennial Library.

Lansky, Vicki. *101 Ways to Say I Love You.* 1991. Fireside.

Lerner, Harriet G. *The Dance of Anger: A Woman's Guide to Changing the Patterns of Intimate Relationships.* 1997. HarperTrade.

Moran, Victoria. *Creating a Charmed Life: Sensible, Spiritual Secrets Every Busy Woman Should Know.* 1999. HarperCollins Publishers, Inc.

Moran, Victoria. *Shelter for the Spirit: Create Your Own Haven in a Hectic World.* 1998. HarperTrade.

Morgenstern, Julie. *Organizing from the Inside Out: The Foolproof System for Organizing Your Home, Your Office and Your Life.* 1998. Henry Holt & Company, Inc.

Sark. *Living Juicy: Daily Morsels for Your Creative Soul.* 1994. Celestial Arts.

Shaevitz, Marjorie Hanson. *The Confident Woman.* 1999. Crown Publishing Group.

Stein, Shifra. *Unlocking the Power Within: Journaling for Personal and Professional Growth.* 1996. Shifra Stein and Associates.

Tavris, Carol. *Anger: The Misunderstood Emotion.* 1989. Touchstone Books.

Karen Rowinsky

About the Author

Karen Rowinsky is a professional speaker, author, consultant, entrepreneur, daughter, sister, friend, wife, mother of two young adults, and stepmother of two adolescent girls, sometimes all in one day! Through her company *Come Alive!* she works with organizations who want enthusiastic members and people who want to create the life of their dreams. A nationally known speaker, she provides content-rich, fun keynotes and workshops that allow attendees to grow personally and professionally.

With over 25 years' experience in health education, she has organized and produced community health education programs and award-winning special events for a women's health center, a hospital, and a free-standing birth center. Karen was the President and co-founder of The Family Center in Topeka, Kansas. She has been the director of a teen pregnancy prevention project, a childbirth educator, parent educator, and developed and taught classes about puberty for girls and their mothers. Karen served on the boards of two national organizations: the National Association for Women's Health and the International Childbirth Education Association. She is an active member of the National Speakers Association.

Karen offers practical and creative solutions that address the issues real people face in the real world. She lives with her husband Rick in the Kansas City area. She loves to laugh and delights in the fall of the year, her friends, "chick flicks," eating in restaurants, mountains, and music. After many years of adversity, she is living the life of her dreams.

For availability and booking information, call
866-269-3511

To contact Karen, write to:

> Come Alive!
> PO Box 11606
> Shawnee Mission, KS 66207-4306
> Karen@50EasyWays.com
> www.50EasyWays.com

Karen Rowinsky

Give the Gift of Energy To your Loved Ones, Friends, and Colleagues

Check your local bookstore or order here.

YES, I want _____ copies of *Come Alive! 50 Easy Ways to Have More Energy Now* at $12.95 each, plus $4.00 shipping. Kansas residents, please add 7% sales tax per book. Canadian and international orders must be accompanied by a postal money order in U.S. funds, call for shipping charges. Allow 15 days for delivery.

My check or money order for $_____ is enclosed.

Please charge my   ❏ VISA   ❏ MasterCard

❏ American Express

Name _____

Address _____

City _____ State _____ Zip _____

Telephone_____ E-mail _____

Card # _____ Exp. Date _____

Signature _____

Please make your check payable and return to:

Come Alive!
PO Box 11606
Shawnee Mission, KS 66207-4306

Call your credit card order to: 866-269-3511 (toll-free)
Fax your order on this form to: 913-642-8777
Order on-line at   www.50EasyWays.com
E-mail your order to: Orders@50EasyWays.com

If you would like your book signed by the author, please attach a separate sheet, printed legibly or typed, with the name of the person to whom the book is going.